From Detached Concern
to Empathy

From Detached Concern to Empathy

Humanizing Medical Practice

Jodi Halpern, M.D., Ph.D.

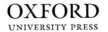

OXFORD
UNIVERSITY PRESS

Library of Congress Cataloging-in-Publication Data
Halpern, Jodi.
From detached concern to empathy: humanizing medical practice /
Jodi Halpern.
p.; cm.
Includes bibliographical references and index.
ISBN-13 978-0-19-511119-4 (hardcover); 978-0-19-976870-7 (paperback)

1. Medical personnel and patient.   2. Medical personnel—Attitudes.   3. Empathy.
I. Title.
[DNLM: 1. Physician-Patient Relations.
2. Attitude of Health Personnel.   3. Emotions.   4. Empathy.
W 62 H195f 2001]   R727.3 H3128 2001   610.69'6—dc21   00-057995

For Rhea

Foreword

As a pediatrician and medical school professor, my clinical work involves the care of children with chronic, often debilitating, but usually non-life threatening diseases. The medical students and pediatric residents who work with me are often frustrated by something about this work and these patients. The diseases are, in some vague but important sense, uninteresting diseases. Usually, there are no diagnostic dilemmas. My patients require care that is relatively low-tech. They need repetitive interventions such as physical therapy, occupational therapy, psychological counseling, and careful nutritional assessments. These can often be performed by non-physicians. The tasks that the residents are called upon to fulfill are not the sort of tasks that they learned to do in medical school. Often, what the patients need from the doctor, as opposed to the non-physicians, is ambiguous or vague.

Year after year, residents "rotate" through the chronic disease hospital, and year after year, I get to watch them struggle with the challenges. Some give up almost immediately. The giving up takes the form of retreating into a narrow technical approach to the care of these chronically ill patients. Such residents stick to careful attention to medications, and remain uninvolved in broader aspects of care. Other residents warm to the ambiguous task of being a doctor to these children. They become involved with families. They want to advocate for their patients in the schools. They get to know the social workers and physical therapists by name. They discuss the subtle frustrations of care plans that have gone awry. I always wonder why some doctors find satisfaction in this sort of care and others don't.

Among other wonderful anecdotes, Jodi Halpern recounts the frustration that Dr. Sheldon Margen felt when he noticed that internal medicine residents didn't seem to like caring for older patients. In particular, they avoided older patients who had suffered strokes. These patients had diseases that seemed uninteresting, complaints that seemed burdensome. These were patients whose diagnoses were already known and so who were of no intellectual interest. The residents gave them disparaging nicknames.

In response, Margen implemented an unusual educational intervention. He designated a time each week when the residents would have to spend an hour talking with each patient. Their assignment? To hear each patient's life story. Halpern notes that, when fulfilling this assignment, the residents "found themselves developing empathy for these patients."

Her use of the phrase "found themselves" is telling in its double meanings. There is a passivity and an almost surprised quality to the residents' experience, as if the empathy that they found themselves developing was serendipitous, unpredictable, and mysterious. How shocking, the phrase implies, that simply listening to an old man or woman talk about his or her life for an hour would lead young doctors to so elusive a quality as empathy! There is also some irony embedded in the phrase, since the process it describes is, on another level, so completely unsurprising as to be almost a natural law. "When one person actually listens to another person's story," Halpern writes, "Emotional resonance and empathy often occur effortlessly."

At the same time, Halpern's phrase suggests that the residents found more than empathy for the patient. They also found themselves. The empathy that they developed was not simply a new sort of sympathy for their patients. It was also an internal quality, a previously unrecognized aspect of their own being. The process of self-understanding is an important part of medical education, often noted by doctors who write autobiographically about their understanding of their own roles but seldom explicitly acknowledged, nurtured, or validated by medical educators.

It is perhaps surprising that empathy for another person is one reliable path to self-discovery. As Halpern carefully elucidates, however, empathy can only start with curiosity and imagination. In order to empathize, one must first wonder what the other person's inner life is like, and that wonder necessarily leads to leaps of imaginative analogies between one's own understandings of the world and the reports we get from others of their inner experience.

There are many different ways to be a good doctor, perhaps more today than ever before. At the same time, there is remarkably little consensus about what a doctor must know, or be, or do, in order to be considered a good doctor. Medical educators, basic scientists, health administrators, bioethicists, patient advocates, politicians, and patients themselves all seem to want something a little different from the doctor. Ironically, this confusion occurs at a time when medicine as an enterprise is more unambiguously successful than ever before. While most people don't know exactly what doctors should be or should do, they seem to have a complex but clear idea of what medical care is and does. And they want more and more of it. But they want it to be precise, quantifiable, scientific, cost-effective. Mastery of medical knowledge and of particular technical skills is the first step down this path. Such mastery is necessary but not sufficient for the type of excellence Halpern imagines.

The challenges facing today's physicians are a different sort of challenge than doctors have ever faced before. In important ways, medicine's success places each individual doctor at a crossroads. Individuals can choose a narrow technical competence or a broader but riskier, more ambiguous, and less definable path towards a more ambitious, less reductionist, and ultimately more humanistic path.

Unfortunately, much writing about this alternative path imagines the choice to be either to stay within mainstream medicine or to leave it behind. In this tightly reasoned book, Halpern lays the groundwork for a different approach. She shows with intellectual rigor that insights from psychology, moral philosophy, and even cost-effectiveness analysis nudge us all in the same direction. Ultimately, high technology and bioscientific sophistication are simply more effective means toward an end that hasn't changed much over the centuries. Now more than ever, doctors need to understand the process by which empathy allows insight into the mechanisms and the meanings of illness for patients. This groundbreaking exploration of the philosophic structure of empathy provides a valuable intellectual roadmap towards a more sophisticated and robust model of clinical excellence.

John Lantos

Preface to the Paperback Edition

During the decade since this book first came out, patients have increasingly asserted their need to be treated empathically. Many medical educators and professional groups want to respond. There is still confusion, however, about what exactly clinical empathy is, and about why and when it is important for medical practice.

As long as practitioners continue to view empathy as an extra step, distinct from the core aspects of medical care, we will see it as something we have no time for. I argue in this book that clinical empathy is not an additional task but rather an adverb, describing *how* healthcare practitioners might do many of the things we are already doing. We can listen to a patient's symptoms with empathic curiosity. We can inquire about a patient's reasons for non-adherence empathically. Practicing medicine through a lens of empathy does not need to take more time, but will increase the quality of patient care and the meaningfulness of providing that care.

Empathy, this book argues, involves both curiosity about and attunement to the patient's predicament. When taking a history, the caregiver who follows a patient's words and non-verbal messages can start to imagine what the patient may be experiencing from the inside-out. The most important pathway to empathy is genuine curiosity and openness to learning something new, something about what another person is feeling that cannot be appreciated just from quickly fitting their symptoms into a diagnosis.

Empathy is a learnable skill when viewed as attuned, curious listening. However, medical practice has not yet absorbed this book's emphasis on *following* the patient's verbal as well as non-verbal communications. Instead of viewing empathy as integrating affective attunement and cognition/imagination, doctors dichotomize empathy into either feelings of sympathy or detached knowledge.

However well meaning, both sympathetic merging and detached understanding lack empathy's value for diagnosis and for developing a therapeutic alliance: First, empathy focuses on the patient's particular perspective—not on emotional or intellectual generalizations. Second, empathy involves acknowledging that you *don't* fully understand how the patient feels and are curious to learn more. Third, detached, intellectual curiosity lacks the resonance with the patient's emotions that guides the listener to imagine how it feels to be in the patient's position. In the past ten years neuroscience has provided a biologic account supporting this book's central claim that emotional resonance informs empathic cognition (Decety et al., 2009). Fourth, empathy often requires tolerating emotional ambivalence. For example, a clinician may be frustrated because a patient neglects her own health. The caregiver needs to accept both the patient's feelings and her own to listen attentively to the patient.

Physicians are not accustomed to following the patient's lead in this way. Instead, too often, medical trainees are taught to say things like "I know how you feel." But ironically, such statements tell a patient that the doctor is not curious to learn more about her distinct experiences. The patient may simply shut down when, with proper encouragement, she might have provided the doctor with crucial information.

Thus, even the training programs that devote significant time to empathy skills miss important opportunities. For example, a model program teaches residents through examples like the following: When a diabetic patient eats a piece of cake and comes in with a blood sugar of 300, the doctor shouldn't scold her, but should instead say, "I like cake too, but here's why you shouldn't eat it" (Boodman, 2007).

Instead, this book argues that it would be much more powerful for the doctor to actually *wonder* what role eating cake plays in this particular patient's life—does she eat socially or does she eat alone for self-comfort?

Empathy then arises as the patient speaks and the physician is moved to appreciate the patient's dilemma—that a more healthy lifestyle would mean trading this bit of love and comfort in the here and now for uncertain future benefits. With this information revealed, doctor and patient can then consider together what other pleasures could be substituted for cake-eating next time, or how to address the underlying sadness.

Clinical empathy is not about acknowledging a shared taste for cake. It is not about seeing oneself as being in the same boat as one's patients, but about being genuinely interested in understanding each person's distinct problems. Compassion and sympathy, while very important, are blind to this difference between self and other. Yet seeing this difference can really improve clinical care. My students in medicine and nursing confirm what others have noticed, that by avoiding statements like "I know how you feel" and instead saying "tell me more," or "tell me what I'm missing," they get much better histories (Coulehan, 2005).

Research over the past decade shows that empathic engagement improves medical effectiveness. Observational studies show that patients give clues before sharing worrisome information (about anything from a breast lump to depression). They check the caregiver's response and then disclose to the attuned physicians much more often than to the non-attuned (Suchman et.al, 2007). Such information is crucial for making accurate diagnoses.

Research also shows that empathy plays a pivotal role in treatment adherence. Empathic communication builds patient trust (Charon, 2001; Frankel, 2004). Trust, in turn, is one of the most important predictors of adherence to treatment (Safran, 1998; Pearson, 2000; Piette, 2005). In recent years, research has also directly linked empathy to adherence and improved patient health outcomes (Beck, 2002; Kim, 2004). Taken together, these and other studies completely upend the assumption that empathy interferes with medical effectiveness.

A concern that this book raises for clinicians is about their own quality-of-life: How can they remain human under enormous time pressures, and how can they empathize without burning out? Increasingly, physicians are dissatisfied with their profession (Zuger, 2004). Importantly, though, research shows that doctors who score higher on empathy measures show more satisfaction and less burn-out (Larson et al., 2005; Thomas et al., 2007). Teaching physicians brief mindfulness practices simultaneously improves empathy and decreases burn-out (Krasner et al., 2009). And doctors are more likely to get tangled in lawsuits, transfers of care, and all kinds of time-consuming and frustrating conflicts if they aren't in touch with the inevitable emotional complexity of providing care. The skillful use of empathy often defuses such problems.

Even if a caregiver attempts to suppress his feelings, he will still hold emotional attitudes that will influence his behavior and cognitions. Physicians who are unaware of their anger can take it out on patients (Halpern, 2007). A clinician who is anxious about his own cardiac risk factors might either minimize or overreact to similar issues in patients.

Caregivers need to take their own emotional temperatures before they advise patients. This book centers around a tragic clinical case. A concerned and sympathetic medical team made serious errors because we failed to consider the role of our own emotional reactions in assessing the patient's prognosis. We were still under the illusion that doctors could be detached rational agents. Over the past decade, research in social and cognitive psychology, neuroscience, and behavioral economics has decimated this illusion. Studies show that detachment is neither necessary nor sufficient for sound medical judgment: not necessary because emotional insights make an important contribution to good judgment overall (Mayer and Salovey, 2002), and not sufficient because even apparently detached medical judgments are rife with inadvertent affective, cognitive, and cultural biases and errors (Groopman, 2007). Detachment in the sense of suppressing felt emotions does not make us more rational; it simply makes us less likely to recognize the inevitable errors we will make. In my current work, I look at how both patients and clinicians better manage health problems when they are aware of their unconscious emotional expectations.

Yet the looming concern about time remains, with increasing demands on what must be accomplished during an office visit. Currently, many doctors are engaged in a clumsy transition to computerized records. Often this means that during the visit, the doctor looks at the screen and not the patient. While such systems may well improve patient safety, the emphasis on recording information during the visit has reduced what little time previously existed for eye contact and non-verbal attunement. Patients report feeling that their concerns are not registering with their doctor "as a human being."

Hopefully using computerized records will become smoother and less of a barrier to connecting. The concern about time, however, is likely to persist. Doctors brought up in the era of "detached concern" still fear that inviting patients to disclose more about their emotional and social worlds will make practicing untenable. They remember the patient who talks for too long. Yet careful research shows that this is not the norm. Direct observational studies show that when doctors let patients talk without interruption at the beginning of the visit, improving their therapeutic alliance with patients, patients spoke for about 90 seconds more (Langewitz, 2002). When, on the other hand, doctors are too hurried, they can miss important problems. The inadequately treated patient then returns, for additional office visits at best and an emergency room or hospital admission at worst. The human as well as financial costs of this to patients, their families, and the entire healthcare system can be great.

Of course, sometimes empathic listening does lead to the disclosure of problems that would otherwise be missed, and which take time to treat. A patient may reveal that she is depressed, or abusing her medications, or subject to domestic violence. Depression is one of the most common reasons patients go to see their doctors, and yet is still more often missed than detected. And, while diagnosing and treating depression may make the initial office visit longer, this problem causes enormous suffering and harm to patients, families, and society, and yet is quite treatment-responsive. Successful collaboration in treating the depression improves the patient–physician relationship, paving the way for smoother future medical care. Substance abuse and domestic violence are more complicated to address, but how can it be good medical practice to routinely miss them? Would doctors and nurses want to overlook multiple sclerosis, lupus, and other chronic illnesses because they cannot yet cure them?

The past ten years of research in fields as basic as neuroscience and as applied as healthcare delivery provide abundant evidence for empathy's role in clinical care. Now is the time for us to challenge the structural factors that increasingly constrain and fragment clinician–patient relationships. The passage of healthcare reform legislation in the United States presents an important opportunity to deliberate about the value of the non-technical aspects of healthcare, including continuity of care. Those involved in medical and nursing education have an additional responsibility to address structural and societal issues to make it possible for the next generation of healers to provide empathic care.

I'd like to end on an optimistic note: The medical and nursing students I teach eagerly adopt the empathy-as-adverb approach. Rather than seeing empathy as an additional challenge or burden, they feel clinically effective and efficient when they connect empathically with patients while doing their core tasks. Through their eyes, I continue to see how practicing with clinical empathy means better healthcare for the patient and a more satisfying practice for the clinician. Caregivers experience the ultimate meaning of their hard work, which is critical in a profession that has been increasingly dominated by externalities (that is, the insurance industry). We know that people find work more satisfying when they are closer to its ultimate meaning, whether they are craftsmen building furniture or physicians and nurses caring for patients. Caregivers need engaged curiosity to see how their medical care makes a difference, not only in physiologic measures, but in their patients' lives. With skillful empathy, physicians and nurses elevate their work from jobs in which they treat disease, to professions in which they contribute to the meaningfulness of people's lives.

Berkeley, July 2010   J. H.

References

Beck, R., R. Duaghtridge, and P. Sloane. 2002. Physician–patient communication in the primary care office: a systematic review. *Journal of the American Board of Family Practice.* 15(1):25–38.

Boodman, S. G. 2007. New doctors develop an old skill. *The Washington Post.* May 15, 2007.

Caruso, D. R., J. D. Mayer, and P. Salovey. 2002. Emotional intelligence and emotional leadership. Multiple intelligences and leadership. In *Multiple Intelligences and Leadership, LEA's Organization and Management Series,* edited by Ronald E. Riggio, Susan E. Murphy, and Francis J. Pirozzolo. Mahwah, NJ, US: Lawrence Erlbaum Associates Publishers, pp. 55–74.

Charon, R. 2001. Narrative medicine: a model for empathy, reflection, profession and trust. *Journal of the American Medical Association.* 286: 1897–1902.

Coulehan, J. 2005. Viewpoint: today's professionalism: engaging the mind but not the heart. *Academic Medicine.* 80(10):892–898.

Decety, J. and W. Ickes. 2009. *The Social Neuroscience of Empathy.* Cambridge, MA: MIT Press.

Frankel, R. M. 2004. Relationship-centered care and the patient–physician relationship. *Journal of General Internal Medicine.* 19(11):1163–1165.

Groopman, J. 2007. *How Doctors Think.* New York: Houghton Mifflin Co.

Halpern, J. 2007. Empathy and patient–physician conflicts. *Journal of General Internal Medicine.* 22(5):696–700.

Kim, S. S., S. Kaplowitz, and M. V. Johnston. 2004. The effects of physician empathy on patient satisfaction and compliance. *Evaluation and the Health Professions*. 27(3):237–251.

Krasner, M. S., R. M. Epstein, H. Beckman, A. L. Suchman, B. Chapman, C. J. Mooney, and T. E. Quill. 2009. Association of an educational program in mindful communication with burnout, empathy, and attitudes among primary care physicians. *Journal of the American Medical Association*. 302(12):1284–1293.

Langewitz, W., M. Denz, A. Keller, A. Kiss, S. Ruttimann, and B. Wossmer. 2002. Spontaneous talking time at start of consultation in an outpatient clinic: cohort study. *British Medical Journal*. 325:682–683.

Larson, E. and X. Yao. 2005. Clinical empathy as emotional labor in the patient–physician relationship. *Journal of the American Medical Association*. 293, 1100–1106.

Pearson, S. D. and L. H. Raeke. 2000. Patients' trust in physicians: many theories, few measures, and little data. *Journal of General Internal Medicine*. 15:509–513.

Piette, J. D., M. Heisler, S. Krein, and E. A. Kerr. 2005. The role of patient-physician trust in moderating medication nonadherence due to cost pressures. *Archives of Internal Medicine*. 165(15):1749–1755.

Safran, D. G., D. A. Taira, W. H. Rogers, M. Kosinski, J. E. Ware, and A. R. Tarlov. 1998. Linking primary care performance to outcomes of care. *The Journal of Family Practice*. 47(3):213–220.

Thomas, M., L. Dyrbye, J. Huntington, K. Lawson, P. Novotny, J. Sloan, and T. Shanafelt. 2007. How do distress and well-being relate to medical student empathy? A multi-center study. *Journal of General Internal Medicine*. 22(2):177–183.

Zuger A. 2004. Dissatisfaction with medical practice. *New England Journal of Medicine*. 350(1):69–75.

Preface to the Hardcover Edition

This book argues that by allowing patients to move them, physicians gain access to a source of understanding illness and suffering that can make them more effective healers. Learning to skillfully empathize with patients is therefore not an ornamental aspect of medical training, but is as critical as learning to perform technical procedures. Although many physicians today believe that empathy increases patient satisfaction with care, the stronger claim this book makes is often greeted with skepticism. Despite increasing evidence that emotional interactions play a role in healing, we still picture medical effectiveness as relying on technical expertise and progress in science. That picture still influences medical students to strive for emotional detachment as it influenced me over fifteen years ago.

I did my third year medicine rotation at a Veterans Administration Hospital during the mid 1980s. The VA is a place where time moved slowly enough for me to learn about my patients' families and outside interests. One patient, Mr. K., had severe congestive heart failure though only in his early fifties. Despite this, he was good humored and outgoing, bolstered by daily visits from his wife who spoke of finally having time with him now that he needed to retire. After Mr. K was in the hospital for several weeks, the attending physician told me that Mr. K was stable enough to go home, but that he needed to be extremely careful about his salt and fluid intake. The team sent me to prepare Mr. K and his wife for discharge, and my tone with them was joyful. We talked optimistically about their plans for the future.

That night I was on call. In contrast to the daytime when a student could talk at length with patients, nights on call involved being part of a small team of doctors covering the entire medical center for emergencies. The team focused on doing procedures, and in the spirit of heroics and technology most medical students eagerly anticipated the event of a cardiac code during their night on call. Although I initially found this repugnant, I was now late in my third year and had begun to adapt to team dynamics, wanting to prove myself in this rite of passage. One evening, when the loudspeaker blasted "code blue" I ran so eagerly beside the resident that we were the first two to arrive. It was not until we got to his actual room that I realized the patient was Mr. K. He was a pale, dusky color, with cool skin, and it was evident that he must have been without circulation for a long time, making brain damage very likely. I felt split into two. One part of me resonated with the energy of my team, excitedly putting in lines, pumping his chest, trying for a heroic rescue. The other part prayed that he be allowed to die in peace rather than survive in a terribly compromised state, twisting the promise of his retirement life into a morbid nightmare.

Mr. K died. I went with the resident to talk with his wife as soon as she arrived at the hospital. The resident told her the medical facts, why Mr. K's heart had stopped, how slim his chances had been for long-term survival. His tone was neutral, matter-of-fact, perhaps he was numbed by the night on call. She listened stone-faced. Watching her, I felt grief and guilt for having gotten her hopes up about his future. I guarded against my impulse to start apologizing profusely, since it was obvious that what mattered at that moment to her was losing her husband. She did not need the burden of alleviating my concerns. I did, however, want her to know that I felt affected by his loss. With obvious emotion in my voice I said, "I'm so sorry that he died, right when you thought he would be coming home." She began to cry, and as the resident quickly left the room I sat with her and felt that just sitting made an important difference.

When I discussed this and other troubling moments during the third year with medical residents and attendings, they encouraged me to become less emotionally involved with patients. They argued that detachment was needed not only for doctors to avoid burning out, but more importantly, to provide objective medical care. This made some sense to me. Because of my own emotional involvement perhaps I had been too optimistic in delivering information to Mr. K and his wife. On the other hand, doctors who carried over the detachment needed for emergency procedures to their discussions with patients seemed to miss important cues about what patients were thinking and feeling.

I began graduate studies in philosophy during the same year. The question that I was probing and continue to find difficult to answer is, what precisely is involved when one person attempts to grasp another's subjective experience? Does this necessarily require some form of emotional engagement? Philosophers whose work I studied in my inquiry into the relationship between knowing and affect were diverse, including Descartes, Kant, Hegel, Wittgenstein, Davidson, Husserl, Heidegger, Sartre, Edith Stein, and many recent writers on the emotions. This work convinced me that although emotional involvement introduces risks of error, there is an important place for subjective, or experiential knowledge in understanding other people.

With this philosophical background, I returned to full time medicine, first a year of internship then three years of psychiatric residency. During the last years of residency, and then as a faculty member I worked as a psychiatric consultant. Doctors on the medical and surgical services called me when patients were refusing treatment or were otherwise in conflict with the team. In these already difficult situations physicians often lack awareness of their emotional reactions to patients, making things worse. This costs more time and effort and interferes with patient care. This lack of awareness was not rigid however, as even during brief consultations physicians invited to reflect on their emotions were able to do so and to shift the clinical problem significantly. For example, the oncology team called to have me evaluate whether the 19-year-old son of a cancer patient should be committed for an involuntary psychiatric hospitalization. He was threatening to shoot the nurses and doctors who tried to go into his mother's room to give her more pain medication because it would make her lose consciousness and he wanted to maintain contact with her. He had no gun with him nor was there any indication that he was obtaining a gun, but his desperation was palpable. His mother was in the throes of dying and he had carried her wasted body into our hospital after signing her out from two other hospitals against medical advice. After a one-hour consultation with the entire team, including the attending physician, residents, intern, nurses, and social worker, the team shifted from hating and fearing this young man to empathizing with him. The physicians acknowledged their frustration at being unable to treat the mother's pain and recognized their various identifications with the case (being sons of mothers, parents of young adult children, etc.). They persuaded the young man to call in his father, who was staying home despite his grief over his wife, because he was overwhelmed by the son's threats. The son asked his father to come in and relieve him so that he could take a brief rest (he had not slept for days). The mother died comfortably medicated with her son and her husband by her bedside, the father later holding the son in his arms.

Repeated consultations like this persuaded me that it was practical for all physicians to learn more about emotional communication, and to use this knowledge to empathize more effectively with patients. This recognition, which went against the grain in the mid-1980s, is now a timely one. In the past few years there has been a shift in medicine towards emphasizing the emotional aspects of the patient–physician relationship. Research evidence from psychoneuroimmunology and other disciplines is showing the power of emotions in healing. Primary care physicians are encouraged to provide holistic care. The topic of empathy is raised more often. Yet, there is no consistent view or in-depth inquiry into what, exactly, clinical empathy involves. Rather, increasing time pressure with the shift to managed care leads to discussions of how to standardize empathy, and how to make doctor–patient communication more efficient.

My hope is that this book's emphasis on developing emotional realism will be useful for busy doctors. After all, missing important emotional cues from patients wastes time, leading to missed diagnoses, inadequate treatment adherence, and inadequate understanding of patients' values in the face of tough medical decisions. Since physicians' own unacknowledged emotions contribute to time consuming clinical difficulties, and a brief consultation acknowledging these emotions can make a big difference, teaching physicians to attend to emotions is more practical than teaching detachment. For these reasons, I envision the audience of the book to include physicians in diverse fields of medical practice, medical educators and students, the medical ethics community, philosophers, and mental and other health professionals.

The book begins with the analysis of a case in which a patient chooses to discontinue dialysis, with the suggestion that the unacknowledged emotions of her medical team contributed to her certainty that her future was hopeless. In the second chapter I look at the modern ideal of detachment in medicine, which coincides with attempts to make every aspect of medical practice scientific and objective by ridding physicians of emotions that might interfere with objectivity. The third chapter examines the characteristic ways that emotions influence reasoning independently of the laws of logic. My argument is that although emotions can lead to errors, physicians can become reflective about such errors and learn to make increasingly realistic emotional assessments. Further and most importantly, by engaging emotionally, physicians can attune to patients' subjective accounts of their illness, linking ideas through imagery and associations, and moods that create contexts. The fourth chapter argues that these distinct emotional linkages are necessary for empathy. Writers on empathy either base empathy in detached reason or sympathetic immersion. Against these models I describe empathy in terms of a listener using her emotional associations to provide a context for imagining the distinct experiences of another person. Therefore, empathy is a form of emotional reasoning, with the risks of error that such reasoning involves. To empathize more accurately physicians need to strive to be self-aware, thus avoiding projecting their own unacknowledged emotions onto patients.

In the fifth chapter I consider the moral implications of the observation that patients' serious medical decisions are influenced by emotional communication with their physicians. The current overarching moral norm is to respect patient autonomy, but in a particular legalistic sense that often translates in practice to avoiding interfering with patients. I argue that the ideal of autonomy is worth preserving, but that the practice of noninterference neglects emotionally distressed patients, especially those who are overly pessimistic about their futures. The final chapter looks at the possible opportunities for healing inherent in many emotionally distressing patient-physician encounters.

This brings the book, and my own fifteen-year inquiry back to its origins. The conflict between performing technically and attuning to patients emotionally that I felt while caring for Mr. K is one that I believe most physicians experience. Physicians are taught that this conflict can be avoided if they cultivate detached concern, a kind of professional humane approach to patients devoid of their own emotional responses.

This book begins by skeptically questioning the norm of detached concern. The inadequacy of this norm requires that we face anew the conflicting role demands on physicians. This work is motivated by the hope that by realistically acknowledging the complexity of their engagement with patients, physicians can sustain genuine empathy for patients in the challenging circumstances of medical practice today.

Berkeley, California   J. H.

Acknowledgments

First I would like to thank Helaina Laks Kravitz. She played a special role as an editor of this manuscript throughout critical stages of development. She read multiple drafts of the work and skillfully guided me to use the clearest language possible to unpack the dense layering of ideas in the text. She is a highly reflective physician as well as a writer, whose own appreciation of clinical realities made her an ideal discussant regarding the subtle aspects of empathy explored in the text.

I want to thank several people for reading drafts of this manuscript. Bernard Reginster provided especially helpful feedback on the philosophical arguments throughout the text. Mariah Merritt, Richard Terdiman, Patricia Bennar, Marilyn Fabe, John Lantos, Joanne Deo, Wendy Martin, Susan Brison, Attina Grossman, and Irene Roberson all read and engaged deeply with this work. Each of them served as important critics and reality checks regarding the more subjective phenomenological claims made in the text about the nature of empathy. Sheldon Margen generously read multiple drafts of this manuscript and offered important feedback as well as clinical examples from his fifty years in medicine to ensure the clinical relevance of the work. Simon Lee helped integrate critical research and gave thoughtful suggestions regarding the cultural assumptions implicit in the text informed by his knowledge of medical anthropology, and generously provided project management at the eleventh hour.

Institutional support is critical for a junior faculty member to complete a book and I would like to thank Tom Boyce at Berkeley and Ken Wells and Bob Edgerton at UCLA for helping provide the conditions for this work to be done. I am grateful for the support I received as the holder of the Martin Sisters Chair at the University of California, Berkeley. Much of this work was done during a Laurence Rockefeller Fellowship at the Princeton University Center for Human Values and a Faculty Fellowship at the Doreen B. Townsend Center for Humanities at the University of California, Berkeley. I am thankful for the support and intellectual community fostered by these centers, my colleagues, staff and students in the Joint Medical Program, the School of Public Health and the broader academic community at the University of California, Berkeley.

Philosophers and clinicians as both teachers and role models have inspired me to think deeply about autonomy, empathy, and the place of the emotions in understanding reality. In particular, I thank Karsten Harries, George Schrader, Maurice Natanson, Barbara Herman, Jay Katz, Howard Brody, Judith Broder, Jed Sekoff, Melvin Lansky, and James Grotstein.

On a personal note, I want to thank my mother, Francine Halpern, for listening to me lovingly throughout my life and for her extraordinary sense of humor. I want to thank Phillip Krey for his loving support, and for teaching me, at age ten or so, how interesting it is to listen to other people. I am grateful to my deceased grandmother Rhea Slominsky, to whom this book is dedicated, for her kindness and playfulness, and for teaching me about emotional strength. I thank Robert De Vries for his support while I was finishing this book, and for love that helps me look forward to the future.

Finally, I have been most fortunate to work with Jeffrey House of Oxford University Press throughout the development of this manuscript. He has made invaluable editorial suggestions and his clear vision of this project played a critical role in its completion.

Contents

*From Detached Concern
to Empathy*

ONE

Failures of Emotional Communication in Medical Practice

The Case of Ms. G.

A medical–surgical team at an East Coast hospital requested a psychiatric consultation for Ms. G., a fifty-six-year-old white woman with diabetes mellitus who had just had her second above-the-knee amputation. She had a long history of kidney failure, was not a candidate for a transplant, and required dialysis three times a week. Although she had willingly come to the hospital for surgery, she was now refusing dialysis, even though she knew that without it she would die in a matter of days. She refused to tell the medical team why, so they wanted both a psychiatrist and an ethicist to evaluate her decision-making capacity. What happened next was a disturbing experience that inspired this inquiry into the role of emotions in the patient–physician relationship.

As a trainee on the psychiatry service, I was sent first to see the patient and report back. I walked into Ms. G.'s hospital room and was shocked to see a child-sized, bony woman curled up under the covers, eyes closed, head shrouded, with her back to the world. She was in obvious pain, face tensed and mouth wide open, as if to yell, although silent, reminding me of

Eduard Munch's painting *The Scream*. My first instinct was to run to her medical team and say, "Give her some morphine." But I remembered that one reason the medical team had called for a psychiatric consultation was that no safe amount of pain medication seemed to affect Ms. G.'s pain. "We're giving her enough morphine to keep a large man comfortable," the intern said when he called me.

In view of her agony, the question of whether she had adequate capacity to make medical decisions seemed strangely detached from the problem at hand, like asking if a person being tortured on a rack begging to die has the right to make that decision. What she needed was to get off the rack. But high doses of morphine were not relieving her pain. After introducing myself, I spontaneously started a guided imagery session with her, as is often done with cancer patients in severe pain who find answering questions too uncomfortable. I asked her to imagine herself in a more relaxing place—the beach, for example, to see and hear the ocean, feel the sand and the soft breeze on her skin. Her face spontaneously relaxed, she kept her eyes shut, and gradually her breathing normalized. She then seemed briefly to go to sleep.

I returned a few hours later and found a group of Ms. G.'s women friends talking anxiously outside her door. After telling me they were worried about Ms. G., one of her friends said, "Ask her about her husband, that creep." When I walked into her room, she was again in terrible agony. I began another guided imagery session, and she relaxed and seemed much more comfortable. I waited for several minutes but saw that she was not asleep. Knowing that time was of the essence and that I needed to learn something about her state of mind, I then asked her, "Is there anything besides your body that is hurting you?" Her eyes shut, she began to speak to me for the first time. "Yes . . . but I don't want to talk about it," she murmured, " I just want to go to sleep." I waited silently to see if she would say more. After a long pause she spoke very quietly. "My husband doesn't love me anymore," she began. "He told me that he's in love with someone else. He moved in with her while I was in the hospital. He said that with my amputations and other medical problems, he could never be attracted to me." She started to cry.

Listening to her story, I imagined facing a future in which I was literally cut off at the knees and abandoned by my husband, with no legs to stand on. But before I could say anything, Ms. G. turned to me and looked me in the eyes for the first time. She looked furious, and I felt almost afraid that she would throw something at me or hurt herself. She screamed out, "Why the hell did you ask me to talk about this? I told you I didn't want to talk. I just want to be left in peace, to sleep and never wake up. Making me think about what he said is the cruelest thing anyone has ever done to me. Don't ask me any more questions! Get out of here!"

Ms. G. was refusing treatment and would die rather than think about the fact that her husband had rejected her. Feeling hopeless, I went to talk to her other doctors and the ethicist on the case. Earlier that day, Ms. G. had told her surgeon that she knew she would die without dialysis and that this was her preference. She felt that her future as a double amputee was bleak and knew she would suffer further complications of her diabetes, such as blindness. He had discussed this conversation with the ethicist. When I told them about her husband, they both commented on how alone Ms. G. must feel but said that she was making an informed decision and that we needed to respect her right to refuse treatment. They warned me against my apparent emotional desire to rescue her, pointing out, "You can't take her home with you, so leave her alone."

I then went to meet with her long-standing internist, Dr. L., a man with a reputation for caring about his patients. "Doesn't all this talk about respecting her right to die seem inadequate given how abandoned she must feel?" I asked. "Yes," he nodded, and sighed with resignation. "But think about it humanely. What kind of life does she face now? Wouldn't you want to die if you had lost your spouse, your legs, your kidneys, and faced a future of blindness and other medical problems? Let's not ask her any more questions, let's just make her as comfortable as possible and accept her decision to die."

As a trainee, I needed to consult a supervising psychiatrist about my approach to this case. I told him not only about the patient's situation but also about the medical team's difficulty in handling the case, ranging from the surgeon and medical ethicist's detached emphasis on rights to the attending physician's sympathetic projections. We discussed the fact that only two years before, after her first above-the-knee amputation, Ms. G. had felt very depressed and hopeless, yet with psychiatric treatment had recovered her optimism and energy. She had gone on to enjoy her work as an artist and continue her active social life. Her past recovery gave me hope that with enough support she could work her way through the current crisis. After all, she had voluntarily come in for surgery in a hopeful state of mind before her husband had told her he was leaving her, and her doctors' notes supported performing the surgery, implying that she had years of reasonable health and functioning ahead. Surely her reaction to this catastrophic news was severely restricting her current view of her future.

The senior psychiatrist agreed that this was probably true but said that we could do little for Ms. G. this time because of the ethical obligation to respect her right to refuse treatment. She was adamantly refusing both psychiatric treatment and dialysis. In his view the long-term success of these treatments required an extensive commitment over time and therefore depended upon the patient's cooperation. Further, the team had tried to reestablish a therapeutic alliance by having Ms. G.'s previous psychiatrist, who no longer lived in the area, contact her, but his call did not change her refusal of treatment. The senior psychiatrist emphasized that no evidence of cognitive impairment had been detected, as can happen in kidney failure patients who have skipped dialysis. He said to me, with resignation, "The decision is hers. She has the capacity to decide, even though she's very upset. Anyway, if we set aside our own emotional reactions, especially our wishes to rescue, it is an objective fact that she faces a terrible future. We need to leave this woman to die in peace and guard against imposing our own wishes on her."

A conference was held with the surgeon, her long-standing internist, the supervising psychiatrist, and the consulting ethicist, and all agreed within minutes that Ms. G.'s decision to terminate treatment needed to be respected. She was given this news as well as more pain medication, and she became lethargic but comfortable for the first time since hearing that her husband had left her. She died soon afterwards, never again speaking the painful words her husband had said to her.

Emotional Irrationality

Ms. G.'s doctors exemplify the difficulty physicians have with patients in emotionally wrenching situations. The medical team, the ethicist, and the supervising psychiatrist sought to respond in a professional way to Ms. G.'s suffering. To avoid judging her situation in an emotional manner, they tried to focus on what they assumed to be objective facts, as if ticking off items on a checklist: Was she cognitively impaired? Did she have the legal right to refuse treatment? Had attempts been made to establish a therapeutic alliance? As if to justify the detachment of the other physicians, her sympathetically immersed primary care internist projected his own viewpoint when he said "Wouldn't you want to die if you were in her situation?" No one on the treatment team ever successfully engaged Ms. G. in a real conversation about her future.

If we accept the traditional medical norm of detachment, nothing seems wrong with the handling of Ms. G.'s case. Although her decision making had tragic results, it was not irrational, because she was able to think in a logical way about her treatment decision. She spelled out her desire to avoid a future of wheelchair use, dialysis dependence, impending complications of diabetes, and rejection by her husband. She pointed out that she had the right to refuse to "process" her psychological distress at her husband's news and that she would prefer to avoid going through such painful reflection. Given her self-awareness and the obvious grimness of her future, her physicians accepted her decision as tragic but logical.

Viewed in this way, Ms. G. was not irrational because she had no primary disturbance in cognition that would suggest that she lacked decision-making capacity.[1] Each of her specific beliefs about her present and future condition, taken individually, was justifiable based on the facts at hand. The problem, however, was that her apparently logical process of justifying her choice to end her treatment—and her life—was, in fact, a defensive strategy to shield her from alternative considerations that she could not entertain for emotional reasons.

Ms. G. was *unable to hope* that she would feel any better once the catastrophic moment passed. The obvious fact that she was terribly upset because her husband had just abandoned her did not figure into her reasoning. The idea of delaying her decision, waiting to see if she changed her mind, had no force.

Although Ms. G.'s decision to die appears to be a reasonable judgment based on her understandably grim view of her future, it was actually the irrational manifestation of a strong, unprocessed emotional state. Her feelings of rejection manifested themselves as a *certainty* that she could never again be loved—that she would be alone and cut off at the knees. Yet her group of women friends stayed just outside her room (she had sent them out) throughout each day and expressed their readiness to support her on discharge. She had felt just as hopeless, they said, two years earlier after her first surgery, but when her depression was treated, she had gone on to love her work and to enjoy her friends. Now Ms. G. seemed unable to feel their presence or think about what they said.

In calling Ms. G.'s view irrational, I do not mean to imply that she was crazy or unique in this irrationality. Rather, a central thesis of this book is that irrational emotional reactions are normal, expectable reactions to sickness and personal loss. Fear and anger are appropriate responses to terrible news. Further, healing involves grieving, a process that includes phases of emotional irrationality. That is, normal aspects of grieving include such irrational emotional attitudes as denial, rage, and bargaining, states that can be considered irrational. Yet it is also generally understood that by experiencing and moving through the transient periods of irrationality involved in the stages of grief, a great deal of healing and realism can be achieved. Grieving, then, illustrates how emotional states can be "practically rational" even when they are not rational in a theoretical sense.[2] That is, irrational, or unrealistic, moments within grief make it possible for a person to arrive at a more realistic emotional state. Though these transient states of mind exhibit emotional irrationality, by fully grieving a person can achieve greater realism. By the end of this book, I hope to show that even catastrophic thinking presents therapeutic opportunity.

Further, Ms. G.'s anger at her doctors may be understood as realistic communication in an interpersonal field. She was subject to intense emotional and physical suffering as well as social loss; she was immobilized in a hospital bed and dependent on the care of able-bodied physicians. The social assumptions of her world devalued her as a disabled woman alone. How was she to reclaim her power in such circumstances? Ms. G.'s treatment refusal may have been the only available way for her to express understandable anger and outrage at terribly constrained options.[3] The problem was that both she and her doctors naively accepted her hopelessness about the future as an appraisal of fact rather than as a strategic psychological response to her situation.

The point of recounting Ms. G.'s case, and of this chapter, is not to describe a rare instance of an extremely disturbed patient, but to use this dramatic, sad case to illustrate how normal people facing illness and loss, and their physicians, can be subject to emotional irrationality. With these caveats, let me characterize the core of the irrationality in question. This analysis may help physicians recognize irrational emotional reasoning in their patients and themselves. Such recognition is possible, I believe, because one can make certain generalizations about emotional reasoning gone awry.

The emotional irrationality in Ms. G.'s case consists of an unwarranted sense of certainty or conviction about reality. A person in the throes of irrational emotion attributes to external reality the grounds for her own interior state of mind. For example, Bernard Lown tells the story of an influential cardiologist who treated a patient with a rapid heart rhythm. She had a low risk of dying but was very fearful, relying deeply on her physician for reassurance. On medical rounds at her bedside, her physician told the treatment team that hers was a case of "TS," an abbreviation the patient took to mean "terminal state." This doctor left the hospital after rounds and could not be located to reassure her that he meant that she had tricuspid stenosis. Nothing anyone else told her shook her conviction that she was in a terminal state.[4] This kind of misattribution occurs with wishful as well as fearful thinking. Another common example is the cardiac patient who starts exercising in the hospital bed, obviously in denial about the significance of being in a cardiac care unit.

Psychoanalysts have discussed the mental activity of selectively seeing concrete circumstances in terms of fears or wishes. Stolorow and Atwood, for example, refer to this kind of selective imbuing of reality with affective meaning as "concretization." They define concretization as "the encapsulation of organizations of experience by concrete, sensorimotor symbols." While they refer generally to "organizations of experience," their cases show how people subject to intense, unacknowledged emotions can attribute to concrete situations their own subjective mental states.[5]

Attributing the grounds of one's emotion to external reality is necessary, but not sufficient, for irrational emotional reasoning. A second characteristic of emotional irrationality is that the person holds her view as an unshakable conviction. Sometimes a person may not even be aware that she feels a sense of conviction. She simply sees things in an absolute way without knowing that this is an emotional point of view.[6] A person who is afraid but is not in a concretized state will view circumstances in terms of their threatening aspect and worry that something catastrophic *might* happen. In contrast, a person with concretized fear, like Ms. G., feels *certain* that something catastrophic will happen. This kind of fear might be expressed, for example, by a middle-aged man whose father died young from a heart attack who is convinced with each bout of indigestion or other chest discomfort that he is having a fatal heart attack. Although he understands intellectually the facts his doctors give to disagree, this information does nothing to modulate his certainty. What most clearly defines emotional attributions as irrational is not error, since, for example, this man could have a heart attack, but unshakable certainty where a certain amount of uncertainty is realistic.

Third, and closely related to this, the emotional belief not only re-sists correction, it does so in a way that is selective rather than being a reflection of brute insensitivity. The man fearing a heart attack rightfully picks out potentially worrisome symptoms—chest discomfort, fatigue, sweating. However, pointing to these symptoms as evidence is a kind of sham justification. To hold a belief in a rational way requires that one hold the belief *because of* the available evidence. To hold a belief on rational grounds does not require that the view be right, but it does involve respon-siveness to evidence. In contrast, a belief governed by an irrational emo-tion is not held based on any evidence, since no matter how the evidence changes, the view persists and the evidence is distorted to justify the view. His doctors may convince the worried patient that the burning chest dis-comfort he experiences after eating a meal is indigestion and not angina. However, he then notices that he is shorter of breath with exercise than he used to be and sees this as evidence of worsening cardiac functioning, just like his father experienced before his heart attack.

Concretized emotions are not only (and not always) out of sync with existing evidence, they also show differential sensitivity to new evi-dence.[7] Most important, this differential sensitivity implies that uncon-scious mechanisms are involved because disconfirmatory evidence is kept out of awareness. This selectivity demonstrates a mental process of notic-ing and yet not becoming conscious of certain aspects of reality.[8]

This kind of selectivity and rationalization constitutes a characteris-tic form of emotional irrationality that influences not only patients, but also physicians, during particularly upsetting moments in medical prac-tice. Sometimes patients respond to bad news, and physicians respond to therapeutic failures, by developing pessimism or optimism that may not seem flagrantly irrational, yet it distorts evidence. Consider, for example, a reported experience in which an intern felt so hopeless after a baby died in the emergency room that he ruminated about how useless all his train-ing had been, sensing that he would never be successful at treating any-one. In his despair he instantaneously felt that all his medical training had been futile, believing at that moment that he "could not even treat a dog bite." His certainty indicates that he was impervious to external evidence, since in fact he had helped patients in the emergency room. Rational feel-ings of helplessness might be expressed as anxiety about being able to help others but would not involve ignoring evidence that one ever had been or could be useful. Although the thought that he could fail any time he tried to save someone is, strictly speaking, logical, his certainty that he would fail is an example of a concretized emotional state.[9]

In a concretized emotional state, the relationship between a person's view and the grounds he finds for it in the world is distorted. Instead of developing a view based on openness to evidence, he fits the evidence to a view. Since the person does not hold the belief *because* of the evidence or reasons, he cannot change his mind based on reasons or new evidence alone.

One particular risk of irrationality, exemplified by Ms. G.'s case, occurs when an entire treatment team participates in concretized emotions. Patients in strong states of hopelessness and fear often evoke similar states in their physicians and nurses, who then behave in ways that confirm the patients' fear. "Projective identification," a term first used by the psychoanalyst Melanie Klein,[10] is a process in which one person's irrational emotions are transmitted to others.

Although psychoanalysts dispute the nuances, the basic idea of projective identification is that a person finds some feelings intolerable and projects them onto other people. This is not merely mental, however, in that the distraught person actually behaves in ways that leads others to take on, or identify with, the projected emotion. For example, a patient who is extremely hopeless about her future may induce feelings of hopelessness in her doctor by presenting only the most depressing aspects of her life. Ms. G. and her treatment team were involved in projective identification. Ms. G.'s suffering was not confined to her interior world, but was expressed through a tortured presence that greatly influenced her doctors. Her concretized belief that her future was hopeless influenced her physicians more than her three positive prognostic indicators—her previous recovery, her vital underlying character, and the presence of supportive friends. Thus, her medical team, too, showed constricted attention related to emotional feelings of hopelessness about her situation.

Ms. G.'s ongoing feelings of abandonment were so strong that she did not feel supported by her friends, doctors, or nurses. Her medical team failed to recognize that she felt abandoned by them precisely because they concretely saw her situation as hopeless. When Ms. G. yelled, "Leave me alone!" she reinforced her state of abandonment. Her withdrawal into a fetal position communicated her rejected feelings to others, despite her own efforts to ignore her husband's message. In fact, the panic her medical team felt in her presence involved *her* intense feeling of being utterly alone and abandoned, despite the presence of her friends holding vigil outside her door and the involvement of the team. Feelings like panic do not affect only one person, they also influence those around that person. I fled her room when she yelled "get out of here." Her doctors were not consciously attuned to her intense fear and did not recognize how they resonated with her anxiety. Otherwise, they might have waited before increasing the morphine and might have found ways of engaging with Ms. G. over the next few days. In various states of sympathy and detachment, they unconsciously colluded in her decision to end her life based on her irrational conviction that she would, in fact, live perpetually in a state of abandonment.

Doctors and patients both have irrational emotions and project them onto one another. Further, emotional communication takes place *between* doctors and patients and helps shape the medical reality facing the patient. This communication is influenced by both conscious and unconscious factors and sometimes leads to irrational judgments and actions. Empirical evidence regarding such factors is being gathered, and interventions to educate physicians to deal more productively with their countertransference, or unconscious reactions to patients, are being developed.[11] The key issue is for physicians to become more reflective about their own emotional responses and learn to use these responses skillfully, rather than try to detach from them and be influenced by them anyway.

Overview of the Book

A central thesis of this book is that physicians' own emotions help them attune to and empathically understand patients' emotions. Even in Ms. G.'s case, I argue in chapters 5 and 6, her physicians' emotional reactions could have been skillfully used to empathize with her and produce therapeutic impact. The risk of irrationality and the opportunity for empathy are two aspects of the same phenomenon of emotional communication.

Chapter 2 begins with the norm of "detached concern" in current medicine. Doctors afraid of making emotionally driven errors strive for detachment from their emotions, presupposing that they can grasp a patient's emotional states objectively and thereby provide more therapeutic influence. Physicians recognize that emotions influence healing. Yet many physicians impose the norm of detachment upon themselves in part because they believe that emotions seriously threaten objectivity, and further, that detachment is the best way to maintain or regain objectivity. They are influenced by the philosophical view that emotions have no cognitive value, a view derived from rationalist philosophers like Descartes and Kant. This view is no longer generally accepted, however, as current philosophers see emotions as playing a cognitive role.

Chapter 3 explores the cognitive role of emotions, noting risks of error and describing how emotions can productively influence understanding. I use the term *emotional reasoning* to distinguish emotion-guided thought processes, such as associating ideas by emotional content, from logical, or detached, reasoning. A central thesis of this book is that logic alone is insufficient for clinical empathy, which depends upon using imagery and associative linkages.

Chapter 4 examines clinical empathy, the practice of which depends upon cultivating emotional reasoning. It explores and ultimately rejects accounts of empathy as detached insight and affective merging. These accounts still divorce emotions from cognition, failing to consider how empathy is a form of emotional reasoning. I develop an alternative account of empathy as an emotion-guided activity of imagination, making use of such distinctive emotional processes as associating, resonance, and moods that provide context.

Chapter 5 focuses on the ethical issue in Ms. G.'s case, the need to respect patient autonomy, and contends that it is both ethically and practically important that patients and physicians cultivate flexible emotional reasoning to genuinely support patient autonomy. Patients in stages of acute grief need empathic support to regain autonomy. To exercise autonomy requires being able to imagine that life is tolerable enough that one can see continuing into the immediate future. Further, autonomy requires having some sense of oneself as an effective agent whose goals can meaningfully influence choices regarding medical care. Yet grief and suffering threaten both a sense of a world tolerable enough to endure and a sense of self-efficacy of even the most minimal sort. Empathy can help patients recover the ability to imagine a livable future. In Ms. G.'s case, if her physicians had empathized with her without fully believing her view of the future, she might have been able to question her own catastrophic emotional prediction.

The final chapter explains what is needed for physicians to develop empathy. It begins with the importance of cultivating emotional openness and curiosity about an individual patient's illness and life experiences. Using the term *curiosity*, however, risks intellectualizing empathic attention, insofar as it implies that it is the doctor's mind that is active and that the patient's emotional life is a kind of subject matter for inquiry. Yet, as Ms. G.'s situation so vividly depicts, doctor's find themselves inevitably enmeshed in emotionally troubling situations, and a mere intellectual curiosity about a patient's state of mind would still constitute a form of denial of the emotional communication already occurring. Rather than scientific curiosity about a patient's state of mind, physicians need to cultivate openness to the painful emotional states that patients communicate *by* having an emotional impact on them.

NOTES

1. Ms. G. was in kidney failure as well as on painkillers, and either could have caused deficits in attention, perception, or logical reasoning. For discussions of assessing patient competency in the context of refusing treatment, see Drane 1985 and Appelbaum and Roth 1982.

2. Theoretical irrationality involves holding beliefs that conflict with the overarching cognitive goal of obtaining truth. Practical rationality is less stringent and requires only that one's views be consistent with one's other goals, which need not include the goal of seeking truth.

3. A feminist analysis of this case would raise questions about the social and cultural arrangements that lead to such situations, and especially issues of power and voice. Patients today terminating treatment are frequently disabled women who are already devalued by society. See, for example, Katzenstein 1987 and Geskie and Salasek 1988. This book's focus on patient–physician dyads is not meant to deny the way medical treatment is socially constituted, an area currently subject to anthropologic and sociologic research. For a critical overview of such research, see Kleinman 1995.

4. In this dramatic case, the patient became increasingly anxious, developed a cardiac arrhythmia, and died. This influenced Lown and other physicians to argue that communication plays a crucial role in treating acute heart patients.Dossey 1991, p. 76–77.

5. Stolorow et al. 1987, p. 132.

6. Marcia Cavell makes this contention in Cavell 1998.

7. A person can hold a view irrationally that, nonetheless, turns out to be correct, as noted in the famous saying "Just because I'm paranoid doesn't mean they're not out to get me."

8. This process of noticing something that one is supposedly not conscious of relates to self-deception, as discussed by Donald Davidson, and "bad faith" described by Sartre. Both Davidson and Sartre describe how the self-deceiver must somehow know the precise things she is deceiving herself about in order to be effective at self-deception. See Davidson 1974 and Sartre 1966.

9. This is adapted from Marion 1988.

10. The concept of projective identification is a complex one described differently by various psychoanalysts. A simplified account follows: One person projects her affect or induces another to feel her type of affect. She then re-experiences the disowned affect through identifying with the other person, but now it is seen as having an external locus, hence alleviating some of her inability to tolerate it as her own. This concept brings to light a philosophic point. Disowning an affect can occur even while one still feels the affect, through the mechanism of attributing it to another source. Therefore, owning a feeling requires more than feeling it, it also involves recognizing that it originates within oneself. See Klein 1952 and Malin and Grotstein 1966.

11. Different patient types bring out marked variations in physician behaviors. Clinicians label certain types of people with whom they consistently interact poorly as "difficult patients," yet there are identifiable interactive factors in such cases. See Crutcher and Bass 1980; Wurzberger and Levy 1990; DiMatteo et al. 1980. Consequently, many general medicine clinicians have sought to recast the label of "problem patient" as a flag signaling an inadequate therapeutic *relationship* that should mobilize the physician to re-examine the interaction. See Anstett 1980; Longhurst 1980; Hooper et al. 1982. In situations in which negative interactions occur, physicians can learn to attend to communication with patients and restore "empathy and objectivity." See Farber, Novack, and O'Brien 1997. In one study of medical students, a high incidence of unrecognized feelings toward patients and potentially harmful associated behaviors were related to impaired interview performance. Medical educators recommend that instructors explicitly address countertransference during interview training. See Smith 1984. In the psychotherapy literature, these issues are discussed under two headings, countertransference and therapeutic alliance. There is currently broad consensus that clinicians need to search out their own patterns of unconscious reactivity (the strict definition of countertransference pertains to physicians' unconscious reactions to patients' unconscious material) to harness their emotions and move toward a more therapeutic interaction. On countertransference, see Racker 1968 and Winnicott 1949b. For a broader psychotherapy approach to therapeutic alliance, see Alford and Beck 1997 and Castonquay 1997. For a more interactionist analysis of emotions and reflexivity, see Mills and Kleinman 1988. Countertransference and the therapuetic alliance in the patient–nurse relationship have been studied intensively. See Morse, Havens, and Wilson 1997b; Morse and Intrieri 1997c; Stein et al. 1997; and Williams and Tappen 1999.

TWO

Managing Emotions as a Professional Ideal

Ms. G.'s doctors were caught in the medical profession's longstanding struggle to achieve an appropriate balance between clinical distance and sympathy. This chapter challenges the two approaches they took—striving for detachment or sympathetically identifying with her—to consider whether emotional communication between patient and physician can become a conscious and skillfully developed part of medical care.

Detachment to Avoid the Errors of Sympathy

Why do physicians, who are increasingly aware of emotional factors in healing, including the influence of their relationship with patients, strive for detachment rather than emotional engagement with patients?[1] Following are some of the reasons physicians give for seeking detachment and some challenges to these justifications. Physicians believe that they need to detach to protect themselves from burn-out as they care for one suffering person after another under great time constraints. Yet, observational studies suggest that physicians are not protected from burn-out by emotional detachment.[2] Detachment is needed, physicians and nurses both assert, to concentrate and perform painful prodedures. Yet even surgeons recognize that performing procedures is only one part of their work and show increasing interest in developing skills for communicating emotionally with patients at other moments.[3]

Another reason physicians invoke is the need to care for patients in an equal, impartial way, not favoring some over others, especially in an era of managed care in which physicians must ration their time and treatments. However, impartiality need not be accompanied by detachment: parents strive to be fair in their treatment of all their children without eliminating their feelings for each child. Yet perhaps the family analogy is irrelevant because physicians today are increasingly caring for strangers in bureaucracies. Not favoring or disfavoring people in these circumstances is challenging because physicians may have inadvertent prejudices toward people with values and backgrounds distinct from their own, and, lacking the time to get to know these patients, may see their needs as less salient.[4,5] Note that this justification for detachment conflates two very different issues, increasing awareness of diverse patient values and the increasing time pressure and bureaucratic structure of medicine. The former demands that physicians develop tolerance and empathy for patients from diverse backgrounds, but it does not require detachment.

To say that time pressure and functioning bureaucratically demands detachment is to draw a foregone conclusion that the patient–physician relationship is of a secondary concern in current medicine. Against this, several research studies are underway showing that even brief contacts with physicians can influence patients therapeutically, both positively and negatively, depending on the physician's empathy.[6] Further, insofar as bureaucratic pressures, including time pressures, make it difficult for physicians to cultivate empathy for each of their patients, this is not a justification *for* detachment (based on the ideal of impartiality), but a sign that structuring medical care to decrease available physician time per patient is problematic.

Although I refer to the "patient–physician relationship" throughout this book, the term *relationship* may be misleading, in that doctors and patients today do not necessarily have the type of ongoing attachment that this word usually denotes.[7] Importantly, this book's arguments about the importance of clinical empathy do not depend on long-standing relationships, nor even on any strong affiliative feelings, between doctors and patients, other than the physician's serious intent to help the patient. That is, this book argues that what makes empathy therapeutic is not the intensity of a physician's positive feelings for a patient, but the ability of the physician to understand a patient's emotional point of view.

We can reject the arguments that attempt to justify detachment as an overall stance to prevent burn-out, permit effective technique, and promote impartiality. We can then focus on the most basic argument physicians give for maintaining detachment: emotions are inherently subjective influences that interfere with objectivity. During the twentieth century, physicians viewed their profession as emerging from a long history of superstition and subjective judgment to be guided by a standard of objectivity derived from the physical sciences. The power attributed to science led physicians to extend the ideal of detachment to all aspects of their relationships with patients.[8] Physicians today uphold a rigorously scientific approach as an ideal for moral conduct.[9] Consider how an American Medical Association Code of Ethics equates "healing," which had traditionally encompassed the art as well as science of medicine, with science: "A physician should practice a method of *healing* founded on a scientific basis; and he should not voluntarily associate professionally with anyone who violates this principle."[10] Physicians are suspicious of their emotional intuitions because they view them as unscientific.

Yet doctors do not deny that much of healing involves understanding and influencing patients' emotions. Rather, the fundamental justification given for detachment in medicine is the argument that it enables doctors to understand their patients' emotional experiences *accurately*, free of their own emotional bias. Renee Fox and Howard Lief, in their classic 1963 article "Training for Detached Concern," described how, from physicians' own points of view, the same detachment that enables medical students to dissect a cadaver without fear or disgust also enables them to listen empathically without becoming emotionally involved.[11,12] Although Fox and Lief were nonphysician observers—one a sociologist, the other a psychologist—their work is consistent with a discussion common to the medical literature of the late 1950s and early 1960s. Physicians attempted to distinguish a special type of detached "empathy" from sympathy. A classic article by Charles Aring in the *Journal of the American Medical Association* in 1958 raised the question of whether empathy is an emotional engagement *between* patient and physician or is a purely intellectual form of understanding patients.[13]

In his article, Aring distinguished empathy, which entails an ongoing separation of self and other, from sympathy, which requires that what affect the patient affect the physician similarly. For Aring, the physician must recognize that he and the patient are not "in the same boat." Rather than feel with the patient, the physician must, he said, remain apart from the "enervating morass of the patient's problems, viewing them detachedly yet interestedly."[14]

Aring wrote: "Appreciation of another's feelings and problems is quite different from joining in them, and in so doing, complicating them beyond resolving."[15,16] Aring's point is that sympathy engenders errors of overidentification, merging, and projection. Think of Ms. G.'s internist saying that her life was not worth living, based on his sense that *he* would not want to live it. It is, presumably, this natural tendency in sympathy to conflate self and other that Aring seeks to avoid in distinguishing empathy, a primarily intellectual act, from sympathy, a way of feeling with the patient.[17]

The tension that persists in Aring's account involves his recognition that even empathy involves some use of physicians' own emotional lives:

> The ability to be empathetic depends largely on the richness of one's own emotional experiences. These experiences are the basis of inner perception—intuition, as it is sometimes termed—the ability to understand one's own feelings and relationships, and by reason thereof, those of others. This view holds that there is no substitute for knowledge of oneself to correctly understand others.[18]

Importantly, while Aring clearly asserts a role for physicians' emotional self-awareness, and even for physicians' heartfelt interest in patients, empathy does not involve having emotional *interactions* with patients. Rather, the physician uses previously accrued emotional knowledge, now intellectualized, to infer what the patient is feeling.

In an influential article written six years later for the *New England Journal of Medicine*, Hermann Blumgart resolves the tension in Aring's argument in favor of detachment. Blumgart described "neutral empathy" as a detached, cognitive understanding of patients' emotional states.[19] Blumgart suggested that "neutral empathy" involves carefully observing a patient's habits and attitudes in order to predict how he will respond to his illness. He contended that whereas the sympathetic physician will grieve for patients and regret his limitations, the "neutrally empathetic" physician will simply do what needs to be done without such reactions.[20,21] This wholescale rejection of emotions, even grieving for patients, may appear uncaring, yet like Aring, Blumgart was, in practice, dedicated to his patients. The severity of the rhetoric reflects the goal of his essay, which is to challenge physicians to rethink a long tradition of sympathetic involvement with patients.

The Tradition of Sympathy

Long before modern physicians believed that detachment was compatible with empathy, physicians believed that being emotionally affected by patients was part of being an effective healer. Just as the tradition of searching for objective understandings of disease motivated the twentieth century interest in detachment, an earlier tradition, dating back to Hippocratic times, emphasized a healing role for sympathy and compassion.[22] Rather than strive for detachment, physicians before the twentieth century traditionally attempted to balance compassion with accuracy by avoiding specific kinds of confusing emotions. The Hippocratic writings, for example, contend that the physician should overcome lust and greed, emotions that can interfere with the practice of medicine. The goal was for physicians to eliminate destructive and selfish feelings and hone their emotions into compassionate feelings that would help guide thinking.

According to the Hippocratic corpus, physicians' capacities to heal sufferers derive from a special *philia* they develop for patients. This "friendliness" is admittedly a purified set of feelings, guided by an impersonal concern for all human beings. Yet, however distant, this *philia* is an actual emotional experience, in which the patients' sufferings move the physicians. The writer of the Hippocratic work "On Breaths" notes that medicine is one of those arts "which to those that possess them are painful, but to those that use them are helpful." The physician "sees terrible sights, touches unpleasant things, and the misfortunes of others bring a harvest of sorrows that are peculiarly his."[23]

While they saw physicians as needing to cultivate emotional sensitivity toward patients, the Hippocratic physicians also foreshadowed the interests of modern physicians seeking to understand physiologia, the *true* workings of nature. In practice, this evolved into the art of diagnosis, literally distinguishing between those complaints and symptoms that are and those that are not relevant to the patient's health. This goal requires physicians to be wary of misjudging the importance of things and of missing valuable information. In contrast to modern physicians, however, the Hippocratic writers did not see emotional detachment as a requirement for accuracy. The accuracy of the physician was based on *physiophilia*, or "love of universal nature, in its special form of human nature."[24] This "scientific," or truth-seeking ideal, was comprised of *both* interest in physiologia and a compassionate interest in human beings.

The Hippocratics' *physiophilia* is one of many ideals physicians have used that incorporate sympathy into effective healing. Other important traditions arose of priestly physicians who had special compassion for sufferers and of gentlemen physicians whose charitable feelings guided their actions.[25] In 1803, Thomas Percival, for example, wrote a kind of gentleman's etiquette for doctoring that he called a medical ethics. He took the characteristics of the ideal doctor to include sympathy, moderation, self-criticism, and understanding.[26]

By the nineteenth century, physicians began to use more familiar psychological language to describe how emotional aspects of their relationships with patients influenced healing. For example, in his 1849 tract on the physician–patient relationship, Worthington Hooker said that the physician sees patients

> in their unguarded moments and when suffering and trials of every variety . . . are acting upon them as tests, searching and sure. He sees much that glitters before the world become the merest dross in the sick chamber; and he sees too the gold shining bright in the crucible of affliction. He sees human passion in every form and condition . . . thought and feeling are often revealed to him unconsciously, and the very fountains from which they rise are almost open and naked to his view, and I may add to his influence also.[27]

According to Hooker, the physician's effectiveness and reliability depend on his affective, or emotional, understanding of human nature. Most importantly, he emphasizes that the physician influences patients therapeutically by interacting *emotionally* with them.

Hooker's ideal physician strives for a kind of clinical distance, or professionalism, in conducting this emotional relationship. First and foremost, he aims to be nonjudgmental. Second, his openness and clarity involve not just emotional sensitivity but also a certain reflective skepticism about his own automatic emotional judgments. He argues that physicians should neither idealize patients through romantic affection nor denigrate them through anger or disappointment upon witnessing their transition "from gold to dross." Instead, the physician's "disillusioning" exposure to human weakness should lead him to a certain emotional skepticism. He will not easily believe his immediate emotional judgments about others. He sees apparent bravery and kindness evaporate under the stress of illness, and he questions his initial responses of respect or affection. Yet the physician does not question the validity of the emotions of respect or affection in general; for, as Hooker is quick to point out, there will be times when such judgments will be borne out, when the "gold will shine bright in the crucible of affliction." The physician cannot see the gold without feeling respect or affection; hence, feeling disappointment is a necessary price for genuinely appreciating patients' emotional experiences.

The function of emotional understanding, according to physicians from Hippocrates through Hooker, is threefold. First, the physician's "heartfelt" understanding helps him grasp the patient's human nature "as it really is." Therefore, within this tradition, the goal of basing medical care on "true knowledge" can be served by a kind of emotional wisdom. Second, by accepting rather than resisting his own emotional range, the physician can stay motivated to take care of patients without resentment, or despair. Third, physicians argue that sympathy plays an important therapeutic role. Within the trajectory of medical thought from the Hippocratic writers to Hooker, the physician's special tolerance of emotions enables an emotional understanding of patients that enhances his reliability and effectiveness.

The Ideal of Objectivity

Yet it is skepticism about the influence of emotions on reliable medical judgment that motivates the modern emphasis on detachment. From the perspective of the early twentieth century, the previous history of medicine was one in which pseudo-scientific practices, such as blood-letting, were ineffective at fighting disease. Physicians found that procedures they once felt hopeful about often did more harm than good.[28] Sympathetic emotions, which were already seen to cause clinical errors, seem to have been discredited as folk practices.

Progress in physiology, microbiology, and chemistry in the early twentieth century offered physicians, for the first time, the opportunity to base diagnoses on an objective understanding of bodily mechanisms. Even before this understanding yielded the improved health outcomes of mid-century, physicians enamored of the laboratory scientist's power donned white coats and wrote of the importance of emotional detachment, severing the link between reliability and emotional depth. They developed tools that allowed them to observe patients with more objectivity and that, at the same time, distanced them from patients. The shift from hearing and touch to arms-length visualization, for example, as well as the use of stethoscopes, helped in creating distance.[29]

Only seventy years after Hooker made the case for emotional understanding, Sir William Osler, the "father" of modern American medicine, extended the new mantle of scientific medicine into the domain of the patient–physician relationship. Osler originated bedside patient rounds at Johns Hopkins University Hospital, in which physicians, dressed like scientists in white laboratory coats, stood before a patient's bed, asking questions like detectives. Osler shared Hooker's interest in understanding patients' emotional conditions in order to influence healing, and he demonstrated that understanding in his own practice.

Osler *himself* made use of emotional interactions with patients in order to be a more effective healer. For example, he cured a girl with hysterical paralysis not by employing some technical intervention, but by recognizing her fear and its role in her paralysis. Yet Osler denied that physicians' effectiveness depends upon emotional engagement with patients. This was because Osler conceptualized healing in a way dramatically different than did Hooker. Unlike Hooker, Osler equated a true knowledge of diseases with overcoming all subjective bias, including all his own emotional attitudes toward patients.

In his 1910 essay "Aequanimitas," Osler emphasized that the physician must strive to control all of his bodily emotions toward patients.[30] Osler argued that physicians can properly distinguish "real" from "illusory" emotional events in patients only by detaching from their own emotions. The goal is not only to neutralize all outward show of emotion, such as blushing or sweating: the doctor must also control the interaction of his mind and body, so that his " blood vessels don't constrict and his heart rate remains steady when he sees terrible sights."[31] Osler takes the physical state of "imperturbability" to be a necessary condition for the mental state of "equanimity." Osler's equanimity is, however, a complex state, arising not from pure thought but from an emotional recognition that physician and patient share a common human vulnerability:

> The more closely we [the physicians] study their [the patient's] little foibles, of one sort or another in the *inner life* which we *see*, the more surely is the conviction borne in upon us of the likeness of their weakness to our own. This similarity would be intolerable if a happy egotism did not often render us forgetful of it. Hence the need of an infinite patience and of an ever-tender charity toward these fellow-creatures (italics added).[32]

According to Osler, physicians, paradoxically, *need* equanimity to defend themselves against witnessing not only the hidden weaknesses of others but also their own hidden weaknesses. Physicians see human frailties that most people never see, even on introspection.

Osler goes on to describe how, from the standpoint of equanimity, the detached physician can "see into" the patient's "inner life." This picture of what it means to understand a patient differs from Hooker's. Hooker did not ascribe to physicians a theoretical understanding of human nature independent of their experiential responses to patients. Rather, he pictured the physician's understanding of the patient as practical: the physician "knows how" the patient feels because of his capacity to grasp imaginatively a variety of affective attitudes. The physician develops a special ability to recognize the expressions of human feeling. He learns to grasp what the patient shows indirectly in gestures and words, even when the patient himself is "unconscious," or unaware, of his own emotion.

When Osler says that the physician can "see into" the patient's "inner life," he presupposes that the physician can set before his "mind's eye" a representation of the patient's psychological life that is fully independent of the observer's perspective.[33] Osler thus extends the ideal of "objectivity," which had already shown its utility in the understanding of disease processes, to physicians' observations of patients' emotional lives. Extending this ideal into the emotional realm involves two assumptions: first, that a physician can be free of bias, that is, free of his situatedness.[34] Second, and more central to this book, he assumes that a patient's emotions are best observed from a neutral physician's perspective—that a physician can see most clearly how a patient feels when he is not moved or affected.

However, Osler also recognizes that physicians are human and will never achieve full equanimity. That is, rather than read Osler's recommendations as a factual description of his practice, we might see his rhetoric as promoting a certain ideal while acknowledging that the ideal is unattainable. His use of the term "happy egotism" is ironic. Osler recognized that detachment is motivated in part by a kind of pride or narcissism. This phrase underscores the irony of expecting physicians to carry on authoritatively as if they were somehow immune from feelings. Osler is aware of the emotional vulnerabilities of physicians as well as patients. Yet his account, influenced by traditional negative views of emotions, fails to address how the common emotional sensitivities of physician and patient can add something to history-taking and clinical judgment.

Osler's model of equanimity and his medical practice contradict each other in several ways. He is described as having a strong personality that had a great positive impact on his patients (and students).[35] Osler's practice involved using his own emotional capacities, and not just objective reason, to influence patients emotionally.[36] Yet his theory cannot accommodate his own therapeutic influence on patients.

Despite his own practice, Osler's rhetoric promotes the idea that detachment serves rationality. He argues both that emotional ways of viewing the world are generally unreliable and that there is no knowledge gained in inhabiting emotional points of view. No meaningful way exists to compare emotional perspectives for their accuracy or appropriateness to a person's circumstances, because the only reliable facts about humans are objective facts about bodies as things.

Detachment as an ideal has an association in doctors' minds with the need for stoicism to shoulder responsibilities in life and death situations.[37] Osler's biography is an exemplar of this ideal of stoicism, in that he frequently experienced the deaths of people he cared for, both personally and professionally. When his own daughter died, he carefully hid his intense grief and quickly carried on with his work.[38] Perhaps his detachment and use of irony are emblematic of the modern physician's self-denial of the "luxury" of grieving and the subsequent disillusionment that arises from dealing with death too mechanically. Medical students describe feeling numb when they begin dissecting cadavers. Residents, too, are expected not to react emotionally when they attend an autopsy of a patient for whom they cared and watch the corpse being dissected. This event is infrequent in residencies today (except pathology) but was part of daily practice in Osler's day. His exhortation to avoid *illusory* positive feelings seems like an expression of his own disillusionment, seeing patients stripped of their humanity during an autopsy.

Osler's views, despite being a hundred years old, are relevant to current physicians. He believed that physicians needed sensitivity to patients' emotional problems, yet he believed that practicing medicine required overarching detachment. His solution to these conflicting demands was to theorize that by neutralizing his own emotions, a physician could achieve special insight, that by not being moved or influenced emotionally by the patient, the physician could more precisely influence the patient therapeutically.

In the Oslerian tradition, physicians aim for equanimity, or what Fox and Lief call "detached concern," not only to treat diseases but also to address patients' emotional needs.[39] The ideal of detached concern is justified by the argument that only an unemotional physician is free to discern and meet patients' emotional needs without imposing his own.

This model of unilateral emotional influence, however, denies the ongoing emotional field between patients and physicians. Patients and physicians unknowingly engage in interactive emotional reasoning by choosing the aspects of the patient's problems they pay attention to or ignore, by weighing the risks and benefits of treatment, and by adopting a view of the patient's future.

The presumption that a neutral, standardizable approach exists to meet patients' distress ignores the diverse needs of patients regarding emotional *interactions* with physicians. Exhorting physicians to have a generic, "ever-tender charity" toward "fellow creatures" is inadequate. For example, some people respond best to reassurance, others to acknowledging the legitimacy of their fears, and others to a more confident and authoritative style. For doctors to take on a generic, professional demeanor of concern is inferior to physicians learning to individualize their therapeutic style according to patients' emotional needs. Further, detachment with a veneer of generic tenderness communicates to the patient that the physician finds something about her emotional state either intolerable or pitiable.

Avoiding Emotional Errors

Osler's explicit claim that the detached physician develops a special professional concern for patients is the same claim that Fox and Lief identify as the basis of the conflicted ideal of detached concern. Physicians today are aware of the tension in striving for both detachment and concern, but do not want to sacrifice objectivity for empathy. It is precisely because physicians recognize the powerful influence emotions can have over their judgments that they strive to detach from them.[40] Yet physicians also recognize that genuine emotional engagement is therapeutic and do not want to sacrifice this, either. Hence the push for a seemingly contradictory ideal. Aring, who recommends detachment, also says that a physician "cannot become interested in them [the patients' problems] short of being interested, a state that only the very greatest doctors achieve consistently."[41]

This book takes the dilemma physicians face seriously but suggests an alternative to detached concern.[42] Rather than making every aspect of medical practice conform to the standard of objectivity, physicians can engage with patients at multiple levels. In addition to evaluating data scientifically, they can cultivate empathy, which, this book argues, demands emotional engagement. Because information gained through emotional processes such as empathy is subjective, physicians need to cultivate skills to evaluate subjective information. Surprisingly, little attention has been given to training physicians to reflect on and assess their own subjective judgments. There are two aspects of becoming reflective about emotional points of view. First, an awareness of the characteristic errors of emotional reasoning is critical because such errors influence medicine, even when physicians experience themselves as detached. Second, attending to emotional communication provides a great deal of information and can be directly therapeutic, as I argue in chapters 4, 5, and 6.

Physicians need to recognize characteristic patterns of emotional thinking because errors result from such influences even when physicians are not emotional in the ordinary sense. Although detachment involves avoiding feeling emotion, emotions are attitudes that influence people even when not erupting as consciously felt events. According to recent philosophical thought, emotions are best characterized as dispositions (or orientations and tendencies) to see the world certain ways, regardless of the level of experienced feeling.[43] The importance of this for medicine is that detachment does nothing to address the influence of such dispositions, including some of the following common clinical errors.

Consider how a physician whose father was alcoholic might minimize her contact with alcoholic patients because of her resentment. A physician who feels anxious about domestic violence might avoid asking patients about this issue. Striving for detachment does not prevent these sorts of errors. Physicians can avoid emotionality by avoiding certain patients or certain issues, and yet it is this distancing that is itself the problem.

In addition to avoidance, another inadvertent emotional influence that detaching does not address is lasting emotional dispositions that create bias or prejudice. For example, doctors caring for patients with sickle-cell anemia, whose painful crises do not necessarily correlate with objective findings, have been shown to be influenced by prejudices and resentment toward patients they perceive to be seeking drugs inappropriately and, as a result, have seriously mismanaged the pain needs of such patients.[44]

In addition to avoidance and bias, emotions can lead to full-blown errors of judgment. An emotion is not simply a bodily "feeling," like an itch. It also involves judging, or imbuing the world with certain qualities that may not be warranted by external circumstances. For example, a physician who just lost a patient to cancer may judge that a new patient with weight loss and lethargy is likely to have cancer, despite the patient having given a history more suggestive of depression. A physician who idealized his own grandmother may underestimate the serious signs that an elderly patient is being physically abused by the family member with whom she lives.

Emotions influence not only what one thinks, but what one does and the urgency with which one acts. Fear, for example, involves more than a sinking sensation in the pit of one's stomach or a judgment that one is in danger, it also involves a disposition toward action: someone who is afraid is urgently motivated to escape. Emotional motives may lead doctors to act with inappropriate urgency, as did Ms. G.'s doctors. In less serious cases, emotional reactions may show up as advising patients with inappropriate intensity. For example, if a doctor had an obese father who died from a myocardial infarction, she might recommend overly stringent measures for overweight patients.

These errors do not necessarily occur separately; often, an entire emotional perspective is awry. Consider the following example explored by Jay Katz in his influential book *The Silent World of Doctor and Patient*. Christian Barnaard, intent on performing a successful heart transplant after the first transplant patient died, *urged* a second patient, Philip Blaiberg, to undergo the grueling procedure. Barnaard's motives were inappropriately influenced by his own desire to be the first successful transplant surgeon. As a result, he did not give the patient the time and space to reflect on the risks he would face and spoke as if he and the patient would set forth on a glorious mission together. This shows distorted attention and judgment, in that he *failed to notice* such obvious things as Blaiberg's extreme exhaustion and displeasure in living a medicalized life, one that he would need to continue after the surgery. Most alarmingly, Barnaard *misjudged* by failing to weigh the fact that no strong evidence yet existed for an overall successful outcome, so that Blaiberg faced a strong possibility of suffering a great deal for nothing.[45]

Emotional errors in medicine often show up as cognitive distortions rather than as overt emotionality. As the Christian Barnaard example shows, these errors can have serious consequences. For example, research about medical errors has shown that medical teams who perceive a patient to be dying because of iatrogenic limitations have difficulty allowing the patient to die. This feeling of guilt skews their medical judgment, leading them to delay withdrawing life support, to the detriment of the patient.[46] Also, it has been shown that when doctors see a patient harmed by a procedure or medication with *known* risks, they avoid prescribing the procedure or medication for the next several patients they see, regardless of the usefulness of the treatment for those patients.[47]

Such errors differ from those caused by inadequate information or bad clinical habits. They are best explained as human errors reflective of emotional reasoning: people, subject to guilt, try to *undo* harm for which they feel responsible. They fear repeating such harm and hence avoid the concrete circumstances associated with the feared event. The motives for such behavior are illogical, because in both cases the fact that the doctor is responsible for a past harm has no predictive value in deciding what the next step in treatment should be. Rather, attempts at undoing and at avoiding associated circumstances are medically ineffective, and yet they are pursued precisely because of inadvertent emotional attitudes.

Ironically, if the detachment physicians strive for means avoiding consciously felt emotionality, then it is inadequate for addressing one of the most significant emotional risks in medicine, that of doctors defensively avoiding patients they find distressing. Although physicians recognize that patients facing terrible losses need emotional support, they still behave in ways that are distancing. For example, transplant teams sometimes avoid spending time with patients who have undergone organ rejection or other complications and are dying in the intensive care unit.[48] Psychological studies of physicians suggest that their own unacknowledged fears of loss and death serve as a barrier to emotional engagement with patients facing death and dying.[49] In a direct interview study asking physicians to observe themselves, they acknowledged such difficulties and found talking about them helpful for overcoming such barriers.[50] Patients whom physicians see as difficult people are often those with disorders that physicians find frustrating or upsetting to treat. One study showed that the patients whom physicians most disliked were those who were suicidal and those who had organic brain damage.[51]

All the errors and biases listed above are caused by irrational emotions that occur in *the presence of outward equanimity*. With detachment as a norm, physicians fail to attend to these errors. Detachment does not make medicine more rational; rather, it forces irrationality underground, where it poses as certainty about the future and other irrational assumptions. Detachment is a poor strategy either to help patients overcome emotional irrationality or to help physicians detect both their own and their patients' emotional irrationality.

This book proposes that recognizing how emotions influence judgment is part of a larger effort to cultivate skillful emotional communication in medical practice. There are three reasons for this proposal. First, given the frequency of errors listed here, and the fact that detachment does not address these errors of attention and judgment, it is critical for physicians to account for their own emotional biases. Second, as I argue in the next two chapters, empathy plays a critical role in medical care, and empathy is essentially an emotional skill. Third, I argue in chapters 5 and 6 that even the kind of irrational emotional communication that erupted in Ms. G.'s case can be transformed into therapeutic opportunity.

Emotions and Cognition

Before arguing for the value that skillful emotional engagement contributes to medical care, the basic philosophical assumptions motivating the ideal of detachment need to be addressed. Emotions are seen as impinging on medical judgment in two distinct ways. First, certain emotional states are seen as disruptive to thinking. For example, if a physician became very angry he might have trouble concentrating. Second, and more fundamentally, even calm emotions are seen as unreliable sources of information about the world because they are so subjective.

Let me address each of these worries in turn. The first is that emotions, as states of mind, impinge upon a person's overall reasoning, as, for example, anger can impinge upon other aspects of reasoning. Certainly some emotional states can impinge upon a person's capacity to reason. However, this does not mean that emotions in general are impingements. Yet a long philosophical tradition survives that defines reason and emotion in opposition to each other. According to this tradition, reason must maintain independence from all influences except the force of logical deliberation. Emotions, which are not products of such deliberation, are therefore seen as impingements on reason. This view is built into the definition of emotion as reflected in the *Oxford English Dictionary* as "any agitation or disturbance of mind, feeling, passion; any vehement or excited mental state."[52,53]

This definition does not do justice to the fact that in our daily lives we regularly experience emotions without finding our reasoning disturbed. As one philosopher has argued, even if an emotion *is* a state in which a person is moved or affected by a situation, this does not mean that the emotional state itself necessarily impinges on the person's concentration or judgment. That is, if I am sad about a friend's illness, the fact that she is ill moves me, but the state of sadness does not necessarily affect or impinge upon me further.[54] In contrast, if I become very angry, my anger itself may then disrupt my reasoning.

The second assumption—that emotions are so subjective that they have no cognitive value—is usually associated with Cartesianism. However, Descartes is actually ambiguous on this point.[55,56] A more consistent rationalist philosopher on this point was Immanuel Kant. Kant viewed emotions as mental states composed of complex mixtures of pain and pleasure, and he argued that feeling states like pain and pleasure, in contrast to sense perceptions, cannot be reality-tracking points of view. He argued that, in contrast to sense perceptions, feelings—pleasurable or painful states—cannot contribute to knowledge of objects. "The capacity for taking pleasure or displeasure in a representation is called *feeling* because both of these involve what is *merely subjective* in the relation of our representation and contain no relation at all to an object for possible knowledge of it (or even knowledge of our own condition) (italics added)."[57]

The reason that emotions cannot provide knowledge is not because feelings are perspectival, or experienced by a subject. Perceiving the color red is subjective in these senses because it requires engaging with the object using a faculty of the subject's. Yet we are allowed to infer that the object *is* red because the object has some property that will always elicit red when such a faculty engages so that a normal perceiver will see red. In contrast, two normally constituted people will not necessarily respond to the same object with the same complex mixture of pleasure and pain, or the same emotion. According to Kant, this variation among people means that emotions represent *nothing more* than how particular objects affect particular subjects. Emotions are therefore merely subjective impressions and cannot provide any real cognitive value.

In medical practice, physicians make use of many subjective forms of information. For example, doctors listening to heart sounds depend on perception. However, physicians increasingly seek technology that can objectively evaluate and correct for the errors of such impressions. It is here that Kant's point becomes relevant: in contrast to sense perception, it seems that there can be no objective form of assessment for the validity of interpersonal emotional judgments.

Rather than challenge Kant's claim, that emotions are tied to a subject, let us challenge the unstated assumption that medical judgment should depend only on objective judgments. The fact that an emotional view is not *immediately or thoroughly responsive* to theoretical reason does not preclude a person in such a state from having the *capacity to assess* her state for its rationality or realism.[58] To counteract medical skepticism about skillful emotional judgment, we need to provide some account of how physicians can assess their emotional views for their rationality.

Philosophical views of emotions have changed significantly since Kant, and it is now generally agreed by philosophers that emotions can be assessed for their rationality, or at least some aspects of them can be so assessed. Emotions, philosophers argue, involve both a cognitive aspect and an embodied feeling aspect.[59,60] For example, to be angry at someone includes being disposed to feel agitated and having the belief that one has been harmed or wronged by another.

According to some philosophers emotions can be assessed strictly in terms of the belief-aspect and not in terms of the affective intensity or persistence of the emotion. This yields clear-cut criteria for assessing the rationality of an emotion. This view, call it cognitivism, asserts that emotional judgments can be correct or incorrect insofar as they involve correct or incorrect beliefs. The difference between rational and irrational romantic love is the difference between rational and irrational beliefs about the lover's behavior or character. So if a lover sees good qualities in her beloved because they exist, her loving view is a form of knowledge. It does not matter that the lover feels more strongly than do others about her paramour's good qualities; it only matters that the qualities she attributes to him actually exist. According to the cognitivists, Kant is incorrect to claim that emotions cannot be assessed for their accuracy.

My view is that Kant's argument that emotions are irreducibly subjective is not so easy to reject, in that emotions influence reason in ways that are not captured by extracting a belief at the core of the emotion. Consider, for example, an instance of anger dissected into the belief that one has been harmed, the bodily feeling of being upset, and a desire for revenge. Cognitivism restricts the assessment of the rationality of the emotion to assessing the rationality of the belief that one has been harmed.[61] Insofar as there is a logically consistent reason for someone believing that she has been harmed, the emotion would be rational.

However, ending the inquiry here, as the cognitivists do, ignores the way the intensity, timing, and patterning of a person's emotions influence rationality. Even if the *belief* aspect of an emotion can be stated as a logical proposition, the *person* having the emotion may be subject to irrationality. What if, in the above example, the person's reasons for believing that she was harmed are logical and correct, yet her anger is explosive and her desire for revenge brutal and disproportionate? What if her anger prevents her from seeing that another is genuinely sorry and will not repeat the harm? What if her anger spills over to all people who look like the person who harmed her? For a philosopher interested in the question of when a specific emotional claim is rational, it may suffice to focus on the rationality of the belief-aspect of the emotion. However, this book has a different focus, which is the question of how a *person*, in this case the physician, can be both emotional and rational.[62] For a physician, anger that is overly intense or persistent impinges on medical judgment.

By narrowing the focus to the belief nub of more intellectual emotions, strict cognitivism ignores how characteristic patterns of emotions reflect the rationality of the person having them. For example, consider a physician who is angry with a patient who is late for her medical appointment. His anger, reflecting his feeling of being inconvenienced, is, strictly speaking, reflective of a rational belief that that type of behavior is, ordinarily, inconsiderate. Yet what if the anger is sustained throughout a long medical visit in which the patient gives a complex history, so that the physician resents her demands on his time and subsequently devalues her medical needs. Though his emotions are narrowly correct, they are overly intense and persistent, interfering with his capacity to understand and treat the patient.

Some recent philosophers go beyond the cognitivists and consider how features, such as the intensity of an emotion, contribute to (or detract from) rationality. Patricia Greenspan argues that the bodily and other feelings involved in emotion do not merely accompany the cognitive or judgmental aspect of the emotion, nor are they merely bodily reactions to a detached cognitive assessment. Rather, as Greenspan puts it, emotions are feelings (affects) *about* one's situation in the world.[63] The strength (and, I would add, flexibility and scope) of one's affect therefore must be assessed in judging the cognitive appropriateness of one's emotions.

Precisely because the intensity and persistence of emotions, not just the beliefs they involve, influence medical judgment, questions about the realism of emotional attitudes cannot conform to criteria for objective knowledge of reality. Kant and Osler are right about the irreducible subjectivity of emotional views. Emotions cannot pass tests for objectivity on the model of sense perception transformed into accurate knowledge of things. However, I take the mistake in holding the ideal of detached concern to be the extension of the criteria of objectivity to the realm of interpersonal understanding in medicine. This book argues that in one area, the *interpersonal* realm, emotions are crucial for understanding reality. As the next two chapters argue, empathy cannot conform to the ideal of certainty that guides medical science. The mental work that physicians do when dissecting a cadaver is very different from the processes necessary for empathy.

Rather than reject emotional influences because they are subjective, physicians need to learn to recognize and critically examine their emotional points of view. This is particularly challenging because emotional influences often occur before a person consciously deliberates. Therefore, rather than detach, physicians need to cultivate greater awareness of emotional influences, paying attention to subtle affective shifts in intensity, noticing underlying affective tendencies, and examining other aspects of emotions that are not reducible to explicit conscious beliefs. The next chapter considers a wide range of ways that emotions influence attention and thinking. The goal is to provide a road map to help physicians recognize various aspects of "emotional reasoning," a term that is not meant to equate emotional influence with explicit deliberation, but to include the wider range of emotional influences on attention.

By distinguishing emotional from detached reasoning, I do not mean to imply that the two are truly independent.[64] The goal of this book is to argue for the skilled inclusion of emotional reasoning in medical judgment by showing that emotions influence even seemingly detached beliefs and decisions. For example, although Ms. G. and her physicians thought that they were being factual in assessing her future, their judgments were expressions of intense, unprocessed emotions. Like stage lighting that sets a mood, emotions highlight some things by casting others into the shadows, revealing some aspects of a situation in part by concealing others.[65] I distinguish emotional from detached reasoning in this and the following chapters as a heuristic device for the purpose of examining the distinct contribution of emotions to overall rationality.

NOTES

1. The term *detachment* is used in this text to refer to (attempts to) avoid all emotional states of mind. In this chapter I describe how this specific notion of detachment came into medicine. Note that this use of the medical ideal of detachment is distinct from ideals of detachment that emphasize accepting rather than extirpating emotional reactions. For example, recent practictioners of Zen Buddhism use the term *detachment* to mean allowing emotions to come and go so as not to attach to any particular emotional state. This kind of mental freedom, rather than neutralizing emotions, is in fact closer to the stance that I describe as facilitating empathy in chapters 5 and 6.

2. Physicians are increasingly vulnerable to burn-out, but this has been linked to time pressures constricting relationships with patients in studies of pressured managed care settings. See Arnetz 1997 and Wilters 1998. Rather than detachment protecting physicians from burn-out, detached models of care correlate with lower work satisfaction, which is a precursor to burn-out. A study of five distinct approaches that physicians take to patient relationships demonstrated that physician satisfaction was lowest in the narrowly biomedical and highest with the psychosocial (emotional communication) approach.

See Roter et al. 1997. Significantly, research suggests that the relationship between detachment and burn-out is complex and that, in fact, detachment corresponds to the "adoption of uncaring attitudes," and is a symptom of burn-out. Programs are being developed to help physicians acknowledge and understand their emotions to prevent burn-out. See Deckard and et al. 1994, Belfiore 1994 and Rosch 1987.

3. The literature in nursing addresses how empathy may make it more difficult to perform painful procedures. See Morse and Mitcham 1997a. For an examination of how surgeons' training impacts their style of emotional interaction and communication with patients, see Levinson and Chaumeton 1999 and Sarr and Warshaw 1999.

4. Physicians are aware that they cannot simply like all their patients equally well, yet they need to pay appropriate attention to all patients. As much as physicians need to strive for freedom from prejudice, however, their role differs from that of a judge striving to be fair to all parties, but is rather that of an advocate. However, a new set of pressures are being applied to physicians to balance advocacy with monetary costs to society, creating yet additional threats to impartiality. The conflicts physicians face between providing impartiality and advocacy are being written about extensively in regard to managed care. See Angell 1993.

5. Lantos 1997.

6. See, for example, Bertakis, Roter, and Putnam 1991; Levinson and Roter 1995; Blanck, Rosenthal, and Vannicelli 1986; and Harrigan et al. 1989. See other references on the healing influence of empathy at endnote 1, chapter 4.

7. John Lantos argues that although it is an important question whether, in an era of managed care, we still need relationships with doctors, moments of emotional openness can be deeply therapeutic. See Lantos 1997. Patricia Benner suggests using the words *repoire* or *connection* instead of *relationship*. Lecture, Townsend Humanities Center, University of California, Berkeley, May 2000.

8. Gerald McKenny's recent work presents a compelling argument that bioethical discourse fails to address the purpose and limitations of medical science and technological intervention, having lost sight of its moral antecedents. See McKenny 1997. For essays on the imperatives of science and technology, see Heidegger 1977.

9. The focus of this text is on Western biomedicine, precluding broader engagements with other traditions, for example, Asian medical knowledge. See Bates 1995, Leslie and Young 1982, and Gordon 1988.

10. From the AMA Code of Ethics adopted in 1957, reprinted in Beauchamp and Chidlress 1979.

11. Through many other descriptive writings, Fox makes it clear that she recognizes that this strategy of detachment is problematic in medicine. Fox and Lief 1963.

12. Fox 1998.

13. Aring 1958.

14. *Ibid.*

15. *Ibid.*, p. 449.

16. Aring's account is more complex than a mere rejection of sympathy. For example, while Aring says that a doctor should not allow himself to make common errors of sympathy, such as blaming himself for the patient's disease, his reflective awareness of the difference between him and the patient "should never lift him in any sense above the misery and suffering." *Ibid.*, p. 452.

17. The assumption that sympathy engenders such problems has been challenged by both feminist philosophers and scholars of nursing ethics, who urge distinguishing the reflective use of sympathy from other uses that are more likely to give rise to errors. Patricia Benner, personal communication, January 2000. See also Noddings 1984.

18. Aring, p. 452.

19. Blumgart 1964.

20. *Ibid.*, p. 451.

21. One sense in which Blumgart is correct, in my view, is in noting that empathy, with its aim of understanding another's state of mind, is distinct from altruistic and caring emotional attitudes, including compassion. It is possible to empathize with someone and hate, devalue, or harm them. Consider such examples as the pathological enjoyment of another's suffering (the sadist resonates with and savors the victim's fear). See, for example, Stoller 1985.

22. Jackson 1990 and Jackson 1992. See also Frank and Frank 1991.

23. From the Littre edition of *Corpus Hippocraticum*, (l.VI,90) and (L.II,634), cited in Entralgo 1969, p. 46.

24. *Ibid.* For a general background discussion of the links between Hippocratic medicine and philosophical arguments about emotions and rationality, also see Nussbaum 1994.

25. See Entralgo 1969, pp. 62–64. "One of the essential qualities of the clinician is interest in humanity, for the secret of the care of the patient is in caring for the patient." Peabody 1927.

26. See Leake 1975.

27. Hooker 1849.

28. See, for example, the history of blood-letting in Stavrakis 1997.

29. Howell 1995.

30. Osler 1963.

31. *Ibid.*

32. *Ibid.*, p. 29.

33. Physicians, according to Osler, need to purify themselves to perform diagnostic detective work, in which the physician attempts to "see through" the patient's illusory subjective complaints. A striking similarity exists between Osler's talk of learning to control one's disruptive emotions emanating from one's "medullary center" and Descartes' talk about controlling the disruptive emotions emanating from the pineal gland in *The Passions of the Soul*. See Descartes 1984. The connection between literal and metaphorical vision in physician practice is explored through Michel Foucault's conception of the "medical gaze". See Foucault 1973.

34. Feminist, anthropologic, and other critical scholarship has seriously undermined this assumption. See Harding 1991.

35. Cushing 1925.

36. Bliss 1999.

37. This contrasts with other health care providers whose work is emotionally demanding yet who do not necessarily feel pressures to develop the kind of battlefield toughness associated with life and death situations. Social workers, nurses, and therapists learn skills to stay emotionally engaged with patients while managing difficult emotions.

38. However, when his son died later in his life, he grieved more openly. See Bliss, 1999.

39. See Deyo and Diehl 1986 and Rhodes et al. 1999.

40. Aring, for example, argues that the emotionally moved physician will become hostile in response to a patient who is very dependent. See Aring 1958, p. 450.

41. *Ibid*. This seems to imply some genuine, affective interest rather than a merely intellectual interest in the patient.

42. See, for example, Mizrahi 1984.

43. Wollheim 1999.

44. Sutton 1999.

45. Katz 1984.

46. Christakis and Asch 1993.

47. See Kouyanou et al. 1998.

48. I observed this often during a two-year period of conducting weekly "psychosocial" rounds at the intensive care unit of a medical center with several transplant surgery services.

49. Kvale et al. 1999.

50. Ptacek et al. 1999.

51. Goodwin and colleagues found that physicians' dislike of a patient was significantly correlated with the patient's degree of cognitive impairment or psychological disturbance. The group of most-disliked patients consisted of patients with signs of organic brain damage and all suicidal patients. .

52. *Oxford English Dictionary*; Simpson and Weiner 1989.

53. A deep philosophical rejection of the view of emotions as essentially altered states is presented by Richard Wollheim in his most recent work on emotions. He argues that emotions are dispositions that can manifest in states of mind but need not do so. See Wollheim 1999.

54. See Gordon 1987, pp. 118–119.

55. The Cartesian denial of cognitive status to emotional judgments is not, as it is often portrayed, a simplistic rejection of subjective experience as a source of knowledge, nor is it a simple result of Cartesian dualism, which has long been rejected. Cartesians do not deny that emotions are real events, nor do they deny mind–body interactions. Rather, they see such interactions as outside scientific explanation. Descartes said that if the union (of mind and body in emotion) were not substantial, emotions could not be efficacious, yet they are. For Cartesians, emotions fail to provide trustworthy knowledge of reality because they cannot meet either of two standards for knowledge of reality: logical certainty for knowledge of the mental, and objectivity for knowledge of the physical. See Harries 1973; Harries 1988. In his later work, Descartes's awareness that limits exist to knowing human experience objectively is linked to a discussion of the emotions. Descartes classifies emotions as a unique source of information for human beings. He says that emotions have *subjective* reality: they are really experienced but cannot *represent* reality in the way that objectively verifiable or logically compelling ideas represent reality. In a letter written in 1643, he modifies the list of the basic building blocks of knowledge he had defined in *The Rules* (1628), where he had argued that only notions that could be grasped with certainty by the reflective thinker could be the basis of true knowledge: number, extension, and the *cogito* are examples of such transparent sources of information. But in 1643 he adds the experience of emotions and bodily agency to this list: "Finally, as regards soul and body together, we have only the notion of their union on which depends our notion of the soul's power to move the body, and the body's power to act on

the soul and cause sensations and passions." Emotions are therefore real as modifications of consciousness, even though they are not sources of certainty or truthful knowledge of reality. Decartes, "Letter to Elizabeth, 1643," in Descartes 1970. See Harries 1973.

56. Because of this dualism, Descartes seems particularly problematic for rethinking the assumptions of modern medicine. For example, a central Cartesian assumption is that health is truly a matter of mechanistic functioning and that ultimately medical science can cure all diseases by fixing body parts. When physicians speak as if medicine can be reduced to a physical science, they are being truly Cartesian. However, increasing data showing how emotions influence healing is making such rhetoric less acceptable, and current physicians rarely share this reductionism, recognizing that patients' attitudes influence health outcomes. Some specific aspects of Descartes's account of emotions that do not presume reductionism are discussed in chapter Three.

57. Kant 1991, p. 40. Note that this selective use of Kant to represent the rationalist view of emotions as unreliable cannot begin to do justice to Kant's thought more generally. I return to his conception of autonomy later in the book.

58. Lear 1998.

59. Note that philosophers' views about the relationship between the bodily aspect and the psychological aspect of emotions have changed over time. In the early twentieth century, William James viewed emotions as originating in a bodily feeling, which then caused a psychological response to that feeling. However, Cannon and others have argued definitively against this view by asserting that what specifically distinguishes an instance of anger from an instance of fear is its cognitive content. Both may involve nervous agitation and lashing out, but in the case of anger it is because one judges that one has been harmed or wronged, while in the case of fear it is because one judges that harm is imminent. Yet the point that the judgment, or cognitive moment, is essential to distinguish the emotions does not entail that affective qualities can be disregarded in assessing the cognitive value of an emotion. See Solomon 1998a; Solomon 1998b, pp. 288 and 282. Also, James's views are discussed in Sartre's work on the emotions. See Satre 1975 (1984), p. 23.

60. Since Gilbert Ryle's work in 1949, most philosophers also include a third component, a volitional aspect. See Ryle 1949.

61. Solomon 1998a.

62. Thalberg 1984.

63. Greenspan 1988.

64. The rationalist dichotomy of detached thought and emotion has been severely undermined in recent decades by scholars in the philosophy of mind, feminist theory, anthropology, and neuroscience. They argue that not only emotional judgments, but all reasoning, are influenced by embodiment and social conditions. See, for example, Greenspan 1988, Gordon 1987, De Sousa 1987, and Meyers 1997. In anthropology, see Leavitt 1996, Lutz and White 1986, Good 1994, and Kleinman and Good 1985. For more recent clinical applications of anthropology, see Kleinman, Das, and Lock 1997; Sobo 1996; Guarnaccia et al. 1996; and Cacioppo and Gardner 1999. In neuroscience, see Damasio 1994.

65. In his recent monograph, philosopher Richard Wollheim similarly argues that the role of emotions is to provide a person "with an *orientation* or an *attitude to the world* [emphasis his]. If belief maps the world, and desire targets it, emotion tints or colours it: it enlivens it or darkens it, as the case may be." Wollheim 1999, p. 15.

THREE

Emotional Reasoning

This chapter explores the subjectivity of emotional judgments. A major thesis of this book is that by critically using these subjective sources of information physicians will take fuller histories and engage in more effective communication. However, using emotions in the service of practicing effective medicine requires noticing and addressing the specific risks of irrationality posed by emotions. This chapter argues that the very properties of emotions that create risks of irrationality create opportunities for knowledge, so long as the characteristic ways that emotions connect ideas are recognized and their limitations understood. Some ways that emotions influence judgment are by linking ideas associatively, arising as "gut feelings," showing inertia, and spreading into moods.

Emotional influences can account for the kinds of medical errors discussed in chapter 2. Consider, for example, a physician who sees a new patient in the clinic who complains of headaches and fatigue. When she asks the patient about her home life, the woman says that everything is fine. Yet something about the patient's body language, perhaps an evasive gaze, makes the physician feel worried that something is seriously wrong and yet difficult for the patient to discuss.

A physician who resonates with rather than detaches from the discomfort and yet shows continued curiosity is more likely to help the patient tell her history. Studies have shown that patients usually will not bring up problems like depression or domestic violence unless asked. Close observations of patient–physician interactions show that patients' decisions to either omit or address such areas depend on whether physicians actually are emotionally attuned to their states.[1]

This example suggests the need to develop awareness of emotional influences on medical judgment. There is cognitive value in attending to aspects of reality that a detached physician would miss, even if such direction is *not sufficient* for reliable inferences about the facts. Physicians can and should assess their emotional reasoning. Emotions play an important role in focusing attention and influencing a person's mental freedom and openness. This process permits a wider and more interpersonally attuned set of ideas and thoughts. By critically evaluating these ideas and seeking further evidence, physicians gain fuller knowledge about reality.

This chapter provides a road map to characteristics of emotional reasoning—associating, "gut feelings," persistence or inertia, moods—that create risks of error. Yet the very same properties can be used in a skillful way to enhance realistic interpersonal understanding. This leads, in the next chapter, to an account of clinical empathy as dependent upon emotional reasoning.

Associational Linking

The most important way that emotional reasoning enhances medical judgment is through the practice of empathy. As I argue in the next chapter, clinical empathy has a specific function, or goal, which is to discern the particular meanings that a symptom or a diagnosis has for an individual. This kind of thinking depends on grasping a patient's associative links between ideas and images. For example, a healthy man in his late thirties who experiences chest pain is terrified about dying because this links to his memory of his father dying at age forty. A depressed woman avoids taking antidepressant medication, not because she experiences side effects, but because she sees the pill as a sign that she is crazy. How does a physician grasp these connections? In these and many other cases, the success of medical treatment depends upon a doctor's openness to following the patient's idiosyncratic emotional associations.

What do I mean by the term "associating"? A core insight of psychoanalysis is that, alongside logical thought, we are always linking ideas in another way. Primary process thinking, as defined by Freud, is characterized by linking ideas that have affective, sensory, and experiential similarities rather than logical similarities. Freud argues that such thinking is characteristic of early life, of dreaming, and of slips of the tongue in adult life and exists side by side with logical reasoning.[2]

At the core of the account of empathy to be developed here is the idea that a listener who is engaged emotionally can associate to another person's associations. This claim, that people in certain emotional states can associate to one another's associations, and thereby expand and recontextualize their ideas and images, is one that we take for granted all the time. That emotional states include susceptibility to taking in new images and ideas is well known within the advertising industry—for example, showing a sexy person smoking a cigarette or driving a car powerfully influences what people imagine when they see cigarettes and cars. Being moved by literature involves incorporating a character's experiences in a way that transforms one's pre-existing ideas and images.

Emotional reasoning involves associational linking.[3] This kind of linking is characteristic of empathy. Rather than looking into the patient's mind from a detached perspective, the empathetic physician relies on her capacity to associate in order to link to the patient's images and ideas. In fact, it is misleading to speak of the physician associating to the patient's associations as if the latter were a pre-existing, static set of ideas. Ideally, empathic communication is a two-way street in which the distinct affective associations of individuals interact and mutually shape each other to yield new thought. It is more accurate to think of emotional reasoning as an intensely associating function. That is, certain emotional states open up possibilities for richly associating.

The idea of mutual influence through associating together, however, raises the problem of individual differences among physicians as well as patients and the risk of poor attunement between physicians and patients. Whereas it is possible to standardize a so-called detached approach to patients, it is impossible to ensure that doctors and patients will consistently attribute the same emotional significance to the events that arise in illness and healing.

Insofar as doctors use their own emotional associations to understand patients, doctors' individual psychological histories and defense mechanisms will inevitably influence how they communicate with patients. This unavoidable risk cannot be overcome by matching physicians and patients on any characteristics, including shared life experiences. Differences in personal meanings can exist even between those with similar backgrounds, and those of the same gender and culture. For example, a woman doctor who has had breast cancer will not necessarily anticipate the concerns of each individual patient with breast cancer. Despite sharing the same illness, the physician and the patient will have distinct emotional profiles in a variety of areas, including fear of dying, investment in a certain body image, fear of suffering during treatment, and concerns about personal relationships and financial security. The two will also find distinct words, phrases, sounds, pauses, and looks meaningful or not, according to their distinct individual histories of communication regarding serious matters.

When these differences go unacknowledged, the risk arises of a particular kind of misunderstanding. Miscommunication often occurs in medicine precisely because doctors wrongly assume they know what a patient means. Just as people use common phrases, but what is said is a reflection of distinct, individual minds, emotional meanings involve a common vocabulary, but the linkages brought to specific situations and the patterns of meaning they create over time bear individual psychological imprints.

Popular literature and humor depict the common phenomenon of two people seemingly talking about the same thing but with unspoken misunderstandings based on their distinct associations. A typical joke in a Woody Allen film shows characters speaking pleasantries while their thoughts and associations are broadcast to the audience. Words that have specific romantic associations for a woman have narrowly sexual associations for him. Ignorant of their differences, each of them projects his or her meanings onto the other person's words, distorting reality. Although this makes the scene comical, in medical practice the failure of physicians to recognize that they and their patients have distinct emotional associations can be problematic.

For example, as Deborah Roter and her colleagues have shown, physicians frequently use medical terms without realizing that their words mean one thing to themselves and another thing to their patients.[4] When doctors fail to ask questions to clarify what their familiar terms mean to patients, terrible misunderstandings can follow. A poignant example comes from the pediatric literature. A doctor told a young patient that he had edema in his belly and did not ask the child if he understood what that means. Several hours later, another physician came to see the child and found him terribly upset. She asked him why and he blurted out, "There's a demon in my belly!"[5]

Although, in this example, an obvious error was made, confusing edema and demon, more often miscommunication occurs without such errors. An example of this might be a doctor asking a patient on antidepressant medication whether she has sexual problems, and the patient saying "no" because she is not having *any* sex and has, in fact, lost all interest in sex since starting the medication. In such cases, the issue is the doctor's failure to recognize the personal meaning of the words.

Returning to the Woody Allen example, neither character is correct about whether the topic of conversation is romantic or sexual. There is no meta-perspective from which all emotional standpoints can be synthesized into one "true" way of seeing reality. Therefore, the fact that emotions are shaped by individual psychological dispositions and histories seems to serve as a source of irreducible variation in what here-and-now experiences mean to different people. If the goal is to make every aspect of medical practice, including history-taking and counseling patients, as standardized and predictable as possible, such variation is clearly a hindrance. However, if the goal is to equip doctors with as much awareness as possible of every aspect of patients' situations, the question becomes how can acknowledging differences in emotional associations contribute positively to medical practice?

Recent work by philosophers, including Jürgen Habermas and Jaques Lacan,[6] suggests that difference or misunderstanding is crucial in developing knowledge. Uncovering a misunderstanding creates an opportunity for inquiry and for the possibility of more refined understanding. Physicians can look for such differences and misunderstandings and use them as the basis for further exploration and empathy. Associative linking accompanied by reflection greatly expands the range of human experience that one is able to imagine, enhancing one's capacity to empathize.

In Ms. G.'s case, I had a distinct emotional association to her situation: the upsetting image of her having been "cut off at the knees." If I had shared this image with her, it might have moved her to grieve, to feel empathy for the pathos of her own situation. It is also possible that *my* image might have been either threatening or irrelevant to *her* imagery. In the next chapter, on empathy, I emphasize the importance of attuning to the patient's specific words and images. However, sometimes it is by the physician offering her own associations that she invites the patient to do so, shifting from an otherwise inquisition-like tone of medical interviewing to explicitly affective communication.

As I emphasize in the next chapter, empathy operates through associative linkages. This creates both opportunities and risks for medical practice. Physicians can certainly impose their meanings on patients, as Christian Barnaard did. On the other hand, physicians can conscientiously seek out a patient's associations to medical diagnoses and treatments.

"Gut Feelings"

Another aspect of emotional reasoning, often taken to signal irrationality, is the sponaneity of some emotions. Certain feelings arise almost instantaneously, before a person has time to think or form a belief about a situation. Doctors, as human beings, are subject to such "gut feelings," which may manifest as quick, intense fear or anger. Neurobiologists describe such feelings as having pathways that can sometimes short-circuit reflective thinking.[7] One justification for detachment is to avoid such influential, possibly negative reactions.

Physicians do need to learn to avoid certain intense, spontaneous emotions, such as rage. However, to be open to spontaneous emotion does not necessarily mean that a person will be subject to states such as rage or will otherwise lack the capacity to manage his emotions. The view of all spontaneous emotion as involving a risk of being overtaken or showing automaticity derives from an ideology about emotions that goes back at least to Descartes.

Descartes states that insofar as human emotions arise spontaneously, they have an entirely mechanistic basis. They are like animal emotions, which he views as utterly machine-like.[8] For example, he says that fear of a scary tiger is caused when the tiger's movements act on a person's visual receptors, causing the person to run away. The psychological reasons for the fear have no relevance to this chain of events. There is no causal role for the person's beliefs or his reflective view of tigers. Further, Descartes argues that even complex emotions, however cognitive their contents, are caused by hard-wired biologic mechanisms and, therefore, are out of synch with present reality.

According to this view, all emotions, however seemingly cognitive, are really simple reflexes that cannot self-correct or attune to present reality in a reliable way. Descartes describes emotional irrationality by analogy to other mechanistic errors. He describes a person feeling pain in a phantom limb, a habituated response that does not reflect present circumstances.[9] He also presents the example of a man drinking too much water because of an incorrect signal of thirst, illustrating the danger of relying on habitual embodied feelings.[10] Similarly, Descartes describes how a person can feel joy because her body signals her mind that all is well, when, in fact, this is not the case. For Descartes, the unwarranted joy, like the phantom limb pain and the unwarranted thirst, results from a physical mechanism that is out of synch with reality. It is the Cartesian tradition that takes the automaticity of certain emotions to imply that emotions in general cannot be influenced by reasoning.

Far from being outdated, the issue of the automaticity of emotions is a topic reemerging in recent philosophy. John Deigh specifically considers the kind of reflex-like emotion Descartes had in mind. His example is the fear that a person feels when looking over the edge of a cliff. This fear shows "automaticity" in that it arises with immediacy, prior to reflective thought.[11] Most importantly, a person can continue to feel fear at a cliff edge even when she knows that she is safe (there is a guardrail) so that this kind of fear seems to be on "autopilot." Therefore, Deigh argues, emotions cannot be belief-like, as the cognitivist philosophers claim. If emotions functioned like beliefs, they would shift with new knowledge. Deigh's point is not to view all emotions as simple reflexes like cliff-edge fear, since he views most emotions as more cognitively complex. Rather, his point is that insofar as emotions involve points of view—seeing something as frightening—this is not determined strictly by cognitive factors but by non-cognitive, biologic factors as well.

The implications of this for medical practice are that insofar as physicians are influenced by gut feelings, they are influenced by non-cognitive as well as cognitive factors. However, my view is that this complex basis of emotional views does not preclude physicians reshaping their emotions over time in accordance with the goal of practicing effective medicine. Few gut feelings are as resistant to reasoning or socialization as cliff-edge fear. Consider, for example, an emotional attitude that is seemingly close to a simple reflex, disgust at the sight of blood. Physicians learn to overcome disgust when performing procedures. Yet the same physician who feels no disgust when doing a procedure, might still feel disgust when at home viewing a movie scene with a bloody body. This suggests that physicians do not merely extinguish a reflex when they overcome disgust, rather they go through a cognitive restructuring that guides their change in feeling. For example, in the medical context, blood is viewed as a signal to take action, or as an object of intellectual scrutiny, a physiologic object.

The psychologic, sociologic, and anthropologic literature[12] show how the most seemingly biologically determined gut feelings are sensitive to interpretive contexts. An example used to show this is the way that physicians systematically de-eroticize patients' bodies in order to perform gynecologic and other intimate exams. This recontextualization occurs in part through the setting in which care is provided, with its systematically clinical tone. It also occurs because physicians focus on their motives of diagnosing disease and treating patients. When one becomes a physician, one reinterprets touching people according to these goals, and in doing so, shifts one's emotional reactions.

Awareness of ordinary gut feelings, unchanged by training, serves medical practice. One important contribution is to provide clues to the physician about the unarticulated emotional states of patients. This happens in part through responding to patients' body language. Consider an example (modified from Patricia Greenspan's example) of a physician in an emergency room. While a patient tells a logically consistent story about her symptoms, the doctor may find herself feeling suspicious about the truthfulness of the story in response to the patient's darting eye movements.

Note that this differs from the case of cliff-edge fear in that the physician is, in fact, making a complex psychological judgment, however rapid. That is, reading body language requires making an interpretation, even if this occurs almost instantaneously. To feel suspicious of someone with darting eyes requires reading the person's gestures as a sign of secretiveness. In contrast to the person at the cliff edge who feels fear regardless of whether she views herself as in danger, a physician who did not view this patient as untrustworthy would not feel suspicious.[13,14]

The benefit in using gut feelings is that they provide an alternative pathway to information. Some of the information could be gleaned through asking every patient a long series of questions, but other information, especially about stigmatized and emotional issues that patients are either reluctant to discuss or otherwise not fully aware of, might never be disclosed. The key for using gut feelings clinically is for physicians to avoid mistaking gut feelings for beliefs based on evidence. This is the value of Deigh's analysis—gut feelings involve views that *may* have no cognitive justification. Physicians need to take their gut feelings as suggestive rather than as confirmatory, and use these clues to seek further evidence.

To automatically perceive someone as untrustworthy is not necessarily to believe that the person is (in fact) untrustworthy.[15] Forming a belief requires gathering sufficient evidence. If the physician learns that this patient has a physical impairment that causes involuntary darting eye movements, her suspiciousness should be allayed (unless she has some irrational prejudice or unstated, contradictory or distorted beliefs).

On the other hand, for the doctor to ignore this suspicion because it is merely a gut feeling would be less helpful than to use this suspicion as a suggestion to carefully review the history. That is, it may enhance the doctor's medical judgment to notice feeling suspicious, so long as this feeling is reflected upon and understood to be subject to the physician's own biases and preconceptions.[16] By remaining reflective, the doctor can use her suspicion as a suggestion rather than assuming it to be certain knowledge of reality. This simple example illustrates how an unreflective, or gut, emotional reaction can lead to fuller clinical understanding.[17]

In summary, those emotions that arise spontaneously, or pre-reflectively, have been presumed to be noncognitive because they are not directly responsive to reasoning. The truth in this view is that some prototypes of emotions, such as fear at a cliff edge, do seem to operate like simple reflexes. Yet even these rare reflex-like emotions are not truly blind mechanisms devoid of human interpretive influences, because they can be influenced by socialization, as occurs, for example, in medical training when physicians learn to overcome disgust at the sight of blood. More important, most other immediate emotions, such as suspicion, clearly are highly interpretative and influenced by social and psychological as well as biological conditions. Insofar as gut reactions can be recognized as such and not confused with secure knowledge, there is no reason to deny them a role in medical practice.

An important set of gut feelings in medical practice are those that arise in resonance with another's feelings. The next chapter argues for an important use of emotional resonance in clinical empathy. *Resonance* involves gut feelings that are similar to the cliff-edge type, in that they arise prior to reflective thought and forming full-fledged beliefs. That is, a person can just feel spontaneous joy or fear, as it were, contagiously, in the presence of another person with the feeling. Closely related, but distinct from resonance feeling, is resonance laughter or tears. In both cases, the contagious affect or gesture need not be accompanied by any focused joyful, fearful, or sad thoughts. Michael Basch, a psychoanalyst, argues that gut feelings are a necessary basis for social recognition of others' emotional states, including the kind of recognition needed for empathy. He describes the innate capacity for two people to *resonate* with each other emotionally, prior to any cognitive understanding, as the basis for developing shared emotional meanings that can become cognitively complex.

Basch is one of many thinkers who argue that there is an essential need for biologically entrained, or innate, affect to learn socially shared emotional meanings.[18] Basch bases his view on the extensive research of the psychologist Silvan Tomkins, who argues that emotional responses originate as innate capacities, conforming to stereotypical patterns.[19]

Ronald de Sousa, a philosopher of the emotions, referring to Tomkins's research, argues that people have shared emotional content because resonance occurs during typical, or paradigmatic, social interactions.[20] This begins in childhood, when toddlers learn the meaning-content of full-fledged emotions by responding with similar spontaneous affect to typical situations. Without spontaneous emotional communication, it is unclear how children could fix their attention on salient social moments and learn an intersubjectively valid set of emotional meanings, according to de Sousa.

It is notable that Tomkins (a developmental psychologist), Basch (a psychoanalyst), and de Sousa (a philosopher), thinkers from three distinct disciplines, converge around a simple idea that challenges Cartesian views of emotions. It is because emotions can arise spontaneously, and specifically because of resonance, that we can, as humans, attune ourselves to one another emotionally and develop shared emotional meanings in the first place.[21] In the process of developing and learning, these authors contend, the originally reflex-like resonance responses of the infant become enriched and individuated by the associative context in which they become embedded. What is rich about this view is that biologic automaticity, far from limiting cognition, enables people to accrue emotional meanings that would otherwise not be developed.

In my encounter with Ms. G., I felt spontaneous emotional resonance in her presence, although, for reasons that will become apparent in the next chapter, I did not successfully harness this resonance to develop an empathic appreciation of her specific feelings. Instead of reflecting, I acted urgently on my strong emotional resonance at least two times. First, my strong feelings of discomfort on seeing her in pain led me to immediately start a guided imagery session to provide some comfort for her, a move that seems to have been helpful. Second, when she became upset with me, I felt so upset that I fled from her room. Perhaps if I had used these urgent gut feelings in the service of empathy, I might have been able to say, in a genuinely emotional moment, something helpful to her about the feelings that were coming up between us.

Note that this example brings together two properties of emotional reasoning, the spontaneity of gut feelings and the associative openness of emotional dispositions, that are essential for empathy. As I argue in the next chapter, empathy involves one person resonating pre-reflectively, with subtle emotional shifts in another person. Gut feelings are the embodied aspect of one person associating to another person's associations. Resonance is not sufficient for empathy, but it is a helpful starting point.

Emotional Inertia

On the other end of the temporal spectrum from gut feelings, which are characterized by spontaneity, are emotions that show "inertia," or resistance to change.[22] In these cases, affect lags behind belief. Physicians sometimes have persisting emotional attitudes that conflict strongly with their better judgments. This can cause harm to patients. For example, white physicians are more fearful of young African-American men with psychotic symptoms, and prescribe overly aggressive treatments accordingly.[23] What is the most effective way for physicians to address destructive inertial feelings?

Consider for example, a physician who feels disgust toward homosexuals, and does not approve of his own feelings. According to the detachment norm, if the physician does not actually hold any false beliefs about homosexual patients, his affect should not get in the way of practicing medicine rationally.[24] However, this presumes that so long as one's detached thinking is logical and based on accurate information, one's lingering feelings have no cognitive influence. Cheshire Calhoun, a philosopher, argues that to have feelings that one does not endorse does not make one irrational. She describes someone raised to be homophobic who grows up and comes to believe that all her assumptions about homosexuals are wrong and yet still feels disgust when a friend tells her that he is homosexual. Calhoun says that in this case, the feelings are like an optical distortion that a person knows is inaccurate. The woman's disgust is a distorted perception of homosexuality that does not actually mean that she believes that things are the way they seem.[25]

Calhoun points out that the person is not, strictly speaking, irrational, because she does not hold contradictory beliefs; she consistently holds the belief that homosexuality is not disgusting, yet she has affects of disgust without full-fledged beliefs. For Calhoun, the persisting disgust is like an outgrown reflex. However, in my view, a physician who, despite her better judgment, experiences lingering disgust *is* subject to a kind of emotional irrationality. If doctors were to treat their inertial feelings like outgrown reflexes, they would ignore the ongoing unconscious fantasies that give life to such feelings.

The disgust that accompanies homophobia differs from fear at a cliff edge, or even disgust at the sight of blood, in that it is never cognitively innocuous. Sustaining disgust toward a group of persons involves an ongoing psychological and social interpretation of their ways of being in the world. Despite a conscious judgment that there is nothing wrong with homosexuals, the persistence of a seemingly "physical" feeling of revulsion betokens a web of images and fantasies, with corresponding values, regarding sexuality and people's status. Such feelings express an interpretation of the world that persists in imagination even when not believed.

As I argue in the next chapter, empathy requires imagining, and not just logically understanding, a patient's world. A doctor who feels revulsion toward homosexuals is enmeshed in a web of attitudes toward the world that threatens her openness to empathize with her homosexual patients.[26] This creates a serious problem in medicine. It is not uncommon for doctors to experience inertial affects that they would rather not have or that they no longer believe are realistic, as, for example, when physicians feel revulsion in the presence of disfigured patients. This attitude interferes with doctoring and is morally as well as psychologically problematic. It seems clear that even if physicians have no negative *beliefs* about disfigured patients, feelings of discomfort have negative effects on the capacity to empathize with such patients. A part of medical training that is lacking is helping physicians learn to work with patients with whom they have inertial discomfort without distancing themselves from such patients.

How can doctors overcome unwelcome but lingering emotional reactions? Rather than try to detach, an emotionally engaged doctor can more actively enhance her own rationality by questioning her emotional point of view. She can engage in a form of "cognitive" psychotherapy with herself. Despite its name, cognitive therapy is a form of behavioral therapy that works on lingering emotions, not on detached cognition. At the same time, cognitive therapy does not simply recondition a person. It works by having a person actively challenge her emotional views of reality.

Cognitive therapy can alleviate the inertial anxiety, fear, and hopelessness that occur when a person suffers from such conditions as panic disorder, obsessive-compulsive disorder, and depression.[27] How does this happen? Consider, for example, cognitive-behavioral therapy for panic disorder.[28] People who experience panic attacks take their own states of physiologic arousal, such as increased heart rate, to signify impending doom. Often the person already holds the correct belief that she is not actually going to die, yet still *imagines* being about to die, and this image is held with overwhelming dread. Treatment involves teaching the person to induce the actual affective state of panic in a controlled way—for example, by hyperventilating in the doctor's office she then learns to relax her breathing. This is accompanied by learning to imagine differently; rather than imagining that death is imminent, she develops an image of herself as able to breathe comfortably, and she gains increasing mastery over her affects.

As cognitive therapy shows, inertial emotions are not mechanistically perpetuated, but are indicators of ongoing mental life. These affects do not exist in isolation, but link associatively to a whole host of attitudes and behaviors. The most difficult cases of inertial affects in medicine arise when an attitude is not universally inappropriate, but appropriate in some cases and not in others. An important example of this is the guilt physicians feel when their patients suffer iatrogenic harm. Recall from the last chapter that even when physicians know better, they show difficulty "allowing" such patients to die, leading to some patients undergoing aggressive cardiac resuscitation attempts unnecessarily.[29]

What is the most realistic and effective way for physicians to manage such guilt feelings? For physicians to detach from them would be to disengage from a basic human tendency to feel guilty when a person one is supposed to help instead suffers or dies. Such feelings cannot be turned off at will without changing how physicians envision their responsibility toward patients. A central part of being a doctor, historically, has been *feeling* a sense of responsibility toward patients. Recall the Hippocratic writer saying that the physician bears a host of sorrows.

Feelings such as guilt are the price paid for maintaining an emotional sense of responsibility and engagement. Rather than basing medical responsibility solely on a bureaucratic sense of duty that would, presumably, extract no emotional price, physicians are guided by an emotional commitment that shows up, in part, as feeling guilt when a patient is harmed by a medical procedure. However irrational guilt over iatrogenic harm may be (assuming no neglect has been involved), this and other primitive emotional attitudes regarding harming or even "killing" patients are the essential shadow side of professionalization.

If we encourage physicians to avoid all guilt feelings, we may thereby encourage them to depersonalize patients. As an extreme example, soldiers manage their guilt for harming civilians either by devaluing the persons they harm or by seeing the harm as the result of a system, thus downplaying their feelings of personal responsibility.[30]

If either of these forms of distancing accompanies detachment in medicine, this would directly violate the single most cultivated trait in physicians, a profound sense of responsibility and regard for each patient's life. A physician cannot achieve a high level of professionalism without developing an emotional sense of concern and responsibility toward patients, and sometimes this generates inertial feelings of guilt. Such feelings, if unexamined and urgently acted upon, can lead to genuine iatrogenic harm, as we mentioned in chapter 2, but the antidote to this is not detachment. Rather, physicians can learn to examine their own inertial affects, to challenge the fantasies that keep these attitudes alive, and to work through their emotions, perhaps by grieving. Even in the case of such troubling inertial affects as homophobia, paying attention to the images and values that accompany such affects, rather than attempting to disown them, is likely to be emotionally demanding yet can help physicians become more open to treating a diverse range of patients.

Moods and Temperament

Another distinct way emotional reasoning differs from detached reasoning is through the influence of mood and temperament. A mood involves a generalizing perspective. For example, in a mood of grief, everything a person sees may symbolize loss and isolation.

Moods create problems for assessing the accuracy of emotional judgment. Recall that according to a cognitivist perspective, one can assess the rationality of a focused emotion by assessing the belief at the nub of the emotion for its accuracy. A belief is true if it corresponds accurately to the matter of fact it addresses. For example, anger at Joe can be assessed for its validity by asking whether Joe, in fact, did something worthy of anger. But the same form of rational assessment is inadequate for moods, a less focused form of affectivity. Returning to the grief example, note that there is no objective matter of fact that corresponds to appropriate grief. If one person feels life to be fleeting and attachments to be fragile, and another takes a heartier view, then who is wrong? The kind of "facts" at stake in assessing the validity of moods are not discrete empirical claims, but such facts as the fragility of human life and the importance of attachments.

Moods are often left out of philosophical defenses of the rationality of emotions because they cannot be reduced to discrete beliefs about the world that can be assessed for their truth content. However, as I argue in the next chapter, moods provide a context for one person to understand another person's emotional experiences. They provide the stage lighting that helps guide attention in empathy.

However, for empathy to be accurate, moods cannot be so general and encompassing that they provide no guidance or constraints on meaning. For moods to provide a reliable basis for interpersonal communication, common cognitive content must exist, despite the apparent lack of specificity of such states of mind. Recall that for discrete, focused emotions, the possibility of shared meanings was linked to common developmental history. According to Basch, Tomkins, and de Sousa, from infancy throughout life, people resonate with others in paradigmatic social situations and thereby "learn" typical emotional meaning. This developmental model relies on the coordination of emotional meanings with observable life experiences, such as the loving touch of a parent.

The problem is that moods are pervasive, subjective emotional states that poorly fit this developmental model. The content of moods does not correspond to observable situations, but to common mental experiences. For example, grieving involves a common mental experience of yearning. However, diverse behaviors are associated with yearning. In some cases a person will talk about a deceased person and want to view his pictures and possessions, and in other cases a person may want to avoid thinking about the deceased and might try to quickly replace him with other people and activities. These are two examples of very different behaviors, but, of course, many other ways exist that yearning, commonly experienced, may manifest in diverse actions.[31,32]

Therefore, using a developmental story does not provide simplified behavioral correlates for learning, as it were, what grief is about. Rather, grieving is irreducibly complex, corresponding not to behavioral facts, but to multivalent social and psychological experiences. Yet grieving does involve shared meaning, as Bowlby, Kübler-Ross, and others point out.[33] Although grieving *behavior* is heterogeneous, some common *subjective* aspects of grieving exist, including disbelief, denial, numbness, withdrawal, bargaining, yearning, despair, hopelessness, acceptance, and resolution. These experiences are not arbitrary; they are reliably shared, although not necessarily in discrete stages and progressions. The example of grief, then, suggests that to understand moods we need to think about the basis of shared emotional meanings in a more comprehensive way than that suggested by the earlier use of the developmental account. Shared meanings arise in emotional development not through correspondence to simple external behaviors but rather in experiences that are socially and psychologically complex from the start.

To take the argument one step further, certain philosophical accounts challenge the assumption that moods are, first and foremost, private, or individual, experiences. One such account is Heidegger's view of moods as shared human experiences in the world. That is, emotions are not interior, private experiences in the first place. Rather, people in the social world are involved in situations that already have a style or mood. For example, people are in a thunderstorm together, and thunderstorms are scary, and sometimes exhilarating. Similarly, social situations are expressive. Another's smile is warming or sometimes too intrusive. This is not to say that individuals do not vary in their idiosyncratic responses to a third person's smile but rather that affective features of experience exist that we do not invent. Moods are not first interior states that are projected onto already-composed social circumstances. Rather, the world is through-and-through an affective world, and our shared capacities for moods allow the world to move us in typical ways.

Heidegger's account suggests a way of thinking about how one person can understand another's moods that is relevant to clinical training. Moods, in his view, are not radically private or interior states that somehow need to be explained to others, but are aspects of shared social experience. Therefore, rather than physicians needing to strive to be detectives who "see into" patient's minds, they need to be emotionally attuned to the moods that accompany the social experiences of illness and healing in the first place. For example, a somber tone is needed to deliver bad news, and a happy mood pervades delivering a healthy, wanted baby. A doctor who attunes appropriately to the style of such moments is, in this regard, more fully attentive to what is happening clinically.

On the other hand, Heidegger's theoretical point should not be overextended, because there are psychological facts that influence medical practice that were not his concern. In fact, patients and doctors are sometimes subject to their own idiosyncratic moods, and these can interfere with listening to others and taking in the mood of the clinical encounter. The problem for physicians is how to be sufficiently flexible and attuned to patients moods. Although, in a sense, the remaider of this book addresses the question of what skills physicians need to attune to patients emotionally, a narrower aspect of this question is how can physicians ensure that their own idiosycratic moods do not impinge upon such openness. One answer is for doctors to be more aware of the impact of their own moods. This is more difficult in some cases than in others. Consider the physician who remarried immediately after his beloved wife died in an attempt to replace her, and never underwent a grieving process. He realized, years later, that he then became intolerant of his patients' grieving processes, urging them to quickly get on with their lives. Only when his second marriage ended and he genuinely grieved both losses did he realize how much he had pressured his patients during those years, sometimes exacerbating their psychological difficulties.[34]

An even more serious challenge to physicians striving for some flexibility and reflectiveness regarding their own moods arises because some moods are so deeply entrenched and persistent that they are states of mind a person can never fully work through or resolve. The intensity, pervasiveness, and endurance of moods vary with the temperament of individuals.[35] Biological factors, ranging from hormonal shifts and periods of neurotransmitter deregulation to genetic conditions that persist throughout life, influence temperament. These biological factors can influence a person's overall affective valence, or tendencies, and can dispose a person to be angry, content, shy, or outgoing. Temperament may also have psychological origins, as has been proposed in models of learned optimism or pessimism, in which individuals systematically generate hopefulness or hopelessness in response to adversity. Physicians of varying temperaments are likely to respond in distinct ways to patients' experiences. Depending on their temperament, physicians may seek risk or avoid it, convey hopefulness or pessimism, or induce calm or anxiety in their patients.

Consider the case of an accomplished cancer surgeon whose story was told in *The New York Times* after he died in a motorcycle crash.[36] His colleagues saw him as an extreme risk-taker. He dared to try experimental surgeries that they would not perform. His fellow physicians described how his intense risk-seeking temperament both served and impinged upon his care of cancer patients.

We know that physicians have high rates of depression and anxiety. We also know that depressed people tend to be risk-averse and that anxious people sometimes overdo things, yet the impact of these states on physicians' decision making has been insufficiently examined.[37] Recognizing that physicians' temperaments influence medical care raises troubling questions. How does knowledge of the biological determinants of mood impact the responsibility physicians have for their own moods while practicing medicine? This is problematic, since people cannot control their own genetic dispositions directly, and moral theory usually does not hold people responsible for attitudes that they cannot directly control. Do physicians owe it to their patients to be aware of their own temperaments and the limitations they at times pose?[38] To the extent that temperamental differences influence specialty choice, physicians already do this.[39] However, even within a specialty, an overly risk-seeking or overly cautious temperament can constrain the emotional flexibility physicians need. At the least, high risk–taking clinicians need to recognize and correct for their own tendencies, as do chronically depressed and overly cautious physicians.

Because temperament is linked to biology, including genetics, it is unclear how far we can expect physicians to go in managing their temperaments so that they will have flexible and responsive moods. For example, increasingly refined medications are being developed to regulate moods. With increased possibilities for managing temperament and mood medically, societal norms are beginning to hold people more responsible for their moods.[40] It is entirely possible that in the near future, this norm will be extended to professionals whose states of mind influence the well-being of others.

On the other hand, if all emotions have an embodied grounding, and if highly intellectual emotions such as remorse and guilt are malleable to thought, then influencing biologically based dispositions through cognitive interventions is possible. This is not merely a theoretical claim, but a fact that is familiar to psychiatrists today, who use biological and cognitive interventions in disorders without regard to theories of causation. For example, whether depression is triggered by social loss or by a genetically determined biological disease, a complex admixture of treatments (psychological, biological, or both together) can be helpful. Further, not only can biological treatments lead to psychological improvement (antidepressants can restore hopefulness), but psychological treatments cause biological change. For example, cognitive psychotherapy for obsessive-compulsive disorder causes magnetic resonance imaging (MRI) changes that correspond to symptom improvement.[41,42]

Nevertheless, alternative psychological models for physicians to manage their moods are needed. One model is Seligman's theory of learned optimism, in which people with pessimistic personalities learn systematically to change the way they interpret experiences so they can feel hopeful in the face of uncertainty and even adversity. Seligman argues that certain aspects of temperament that appear to be biological givens are actually the results of early learning about how to handle defeats, so that some people learn to become passive and self-blaming while others learn to become active and to blame transient circumstances. The relevance of this model to medicine is that it offers a skillful way to redirect moods toward a more realistic and open appraisal of circumstances without denying emotionality and temperament.[43] In contrast to the "power of positive thinking," Seligman advocates not white-washing but challenging unrealistic negative assumptions. In this regard, this model seems compatible with the realism for which physicians need to strive.[44]

The Strategic Nature of Emotions

So far, this chapter has argued that by cultivating greater emotional flexibility physicians can develp a fuller understanding of reality. However, this presumes that emotions themselves, and not just the thoughts we have about them, can be guided by realism. What motivates emotions, and is this consistent with realism? The question of motivation assumes that there is some common goal that emotions strive towards in mental life. This is analogous to asserting that beliefs seek after truth, and that aesthetic judgments are guided by beauty, even though not all beliefs are true and not all aesthetic judgments attuned to the beautiful.

According to one influential account, represented by diverse thinkers including Sartre and Freud, emotions seek to fulfill pre-logical psychological wishes. That is, they not only strive to meet biological needs but are guided by the fantasy lives of persons. The two thinkers, however, spell this out in distinct ways, one of which allows for the possibility of cultivating emotions that are consistent with realism, the other of which does not.

Jean-Paul Sarte presents a view of emotions as literally insulating a person in a "magical" world of wish-fulfilling fantasy. That is, emotions are peculiarly self-deceptive states in which one soothes oneself magically rather than acting effectively in the world (or when such action is impossible).[45] He provides a famous example of someone seeing a threatening stranger outside the window and fainting in fear, thus magically avoiding harm, but, of course, not actually escaping harm.[46,47]

Sartre's view that emotions, in general, are wish-fulfilling states links to some basic tenets of psychoanalytic thought. Psychoanalytic theory, beginning with Freud, sees emotions as serving unconscious needs, although to call these needs wishes in the ordinary sense of the term is misleading. One example of such need involves repeating unresolved traumatic situations, and this hardly pleases a person in the way the term *wish-fulfilling* ordinarily suggests. The point for Freud is that emotions involve primary process reasoning, which is fundamentally impractical and unrealistic.[48] Yet presumably Freud did not share Sartre's conviction that this reasoning can never be influenced by reflection, because psychoanalysis is aimed precisely at shifting one's emotional responses toward realism.

Both Sarte and Freud see emotions as functioning strategically, serving personal needs or goals. For Sartre these needs all involve preserving what he refers to as self-esteem, and describes as a sense of security in one's ongoing self. Sartre describes this strategic function as essentially falsifying reality because there is, in his view, no real or essential self. In contrast, Freud does not see all strategic goals as requiring falsifying reality. Certain narcissistic wishes involve falsifying reality, since from infancy to death we struggle with desires to be more potent and important than we really are. However, psychological maturity involves overcoming the insulation of narcissism, so that one can wish for or want something very much and still be realistic, as for example, when one hopes for a positive outcome but recognizes that the evidence shows it to be unlikely.

The kind of strategic interests that emotions serve are not as narcissistically oriented as Sartre portrayed them as being. Emotions do not necessarily insulate us from others or boost our own feelings of pride. Emotions can motivate a person to care more for another's well being than for her own, as occurs with feelings of parental love. Emotions help us maintain attachments, survive conflicts and avoid harm.[49] These goals seem to require functioning realistically in social relations. This leads to the thought that even if emotions serve strategic needs to maintain one's sense of self, this can still be compatible with seeking realistic interpersonal understanding.[50,51]

One example of this compatibility is certain uses of empathy. Empathy clearly can serve strategic needs by being especially realistic. That is, precisely by reading others accurately, one can be more socially competent and gain self-confidence. Perhaps this example, however, puts the cart before the horse, since empathy is a complex mental activity using emotions in particular ways, as I will describe in the next chapter. A much simpler example, outside of the topic of the emotions, can make the point that an activity can be both strategic and reality-seeking. Consider the activity of learning to move one's body in the world. Developing an accurate sense of one's range of movement and size, for example learning to negotiate narrow passageways, is critical to successful movement in the world.[52] Knowing how to move one's body effectively, which meets strategic needs, depends upon the accuracy or realism of one's body knowledge.[53]

By analogy, in order for emotions to guide a person strategically in the social world, they must have certain accuracy and appropriateness to circumstances. This is especially true when the strategic goal of maintaining the self is looked at over time rather than at a snapshot in time. Over time, one is sure to be subject to feedback from others. If, for example, a person cannot face her mistakes and blames others to preserve her own self-esteem, ultimately her apparently strategic response is likely to backfire, leading to broken relationships and less self-esteem. Sartre's model fails to account for the distinction between those emotions that are realistic indicators in social relations and those that are fundamentally defensive and isolating.

Emotions help us negotiate the social world realistically, and not always by boosting immediate self-esteem. Emotions such as grief and regret involve transient feelings of diminished self-esteem. Yet while these emotions do not soothe the self magically, as Sartre describes, they function strategically toward the development and sustenance of the self. They contribute to one's sense of integrity, attachment to others, feelings of belonging, and non-alienation from fundamental goals in life.

Applying this to medicine, physicians can cultivate their emotions according to their genuine interest in being realistic with patients. However, there are several specific reasons why cultivating realistic emotions may be difficult. First, doctors continually deal with issues people dislike viewing realistically—death, dying, suffering, and loss. Perhaps, in these particular cases, we cannot help but rationalize emotionally out of a need to protect ourselves from harsh reality. Doctors need to be aware of such rationalizations to prevent committing errors of wishful thinking.

Second, physicians are exposed to some of the worst examples of human behavior, including child abuse, domestic violence, substance abuse, negligence, rape, and other terrible acts. Staying emotionally attuned in such cases involves feeling disturbed in ways that may be difficult to tolerate. After developing a caring relationship with a patient, a doctor may find it difficult to recognize that the patient has been involved in some self-destructive behavior. Doctors invest a great deal in idealizing the patients that they care about to avoid such difficult emotions.[54]

Third, medicine is practiced in an organizational environment that can itself create terrible conflicts for physicians. Doctors working in health care systems that routinely under-serve the poor often become emotionally inured to these patients. Doctors in gate-keeping roles sometimes sacrifice realism, honesty, and integrity to maintain emotional homeostasis. The literature is growing on the kinds of organizational structures that serve and disserve patient–physician relationships.[55]

It was within these three constraints that Ms. G.'s treatment occurred. Her physicians feared facing a situation like hers, and they had been trained to detach from or deny, rather than become reflective about, their fear. Her situation was, in fact, terribly hard to face. Further, the physicians involved were working under intense organizational pressures to handle all cases as expeditiously as possible. When Ms. G.'s doctors said to me, "You can't take her home with you, so leave her alone," they were rationalizing. Their belief that further engagement with her would not help her served to relieve them of a sense of burden and responsibility for Ms. G. Yet, in the long term, each doctor probably felt unsettled about her care, so that a better handling of the whole situation would probably have served the long-term strategic interests of all the physicians involved.

In summary, the strategic aspect of emotions does not imply that emotions are unrealistic, nor do they preclude physicians taking a genuine interest in their patients' needs, even when doing so conflicts with their self-interest. A longstanding philosophical tradition, going back to Aristotle, argues that emotions can be educated to express our long-term, socially (in his view, morally) grounded interests, rather than our short-term needs. Aristotle gives the example of deep friendships that engender loyalty that controls one's impulses to gratify oneself at the friend's expense.[56] According to this view, a physician who can tolerate emotions that transiently threaten self-esteem need not possess exceptional altruism but rather has been educated to cultivate emotional attentiveness to others as part of her own long-term success. Physicians frequently describe how developing empathy, in fact, makes their practice more satisfying and sustaining.[57]

This chapter has argued that the very properties of emotional reasoning that traditionally have been equated with irrationality can be harnessed in the service of medical care if physicians can develop self-awareness. The most important use of emotional reasoning is for the practice of clinical empathy. As I argue in the next chapter, empathy is neither detached reasoning nor untrained sympathy, but something distinct, straddling cognitive and affective capacities. By developing a specific account of the mental processes involved in empathy, I will establish a basis for arguing why emotional engagement contributes to effective medical practice.

NOTES

1. Rogriguez et al. And Suchman et al. 1997.

2. Freud 1949.

3. The heuristic of distinguishing emotional reasoning from detached thought is misleading here, because I do not mean to suggest that it is only explicitly emotional ideas that link associatively. Rather, even seemingly unemotional, spontaneous thoughts are often connected through emotional assocations. This is why the psychoanalytic method of free association reveals underlying emotional dynamics.

4. Hall et al. 1999 and Sleath et al. 1999.

5. Perrin 1981.

6. For Lacan, encountering another with a different perspective makes possible "a new mode of cognition or information gathering whereby ignorance itself becomes structurally informative, in an asymmetrically reflexive dialogue in which the interlocutors—

through language—inform each other of what they do not know." From Felman 1987, p. 60. See also Habermas 1974.

7. Dasmasio 1994.

8. Descartes 1984, *The Passions of the Soul*, p. 338.

9. Descartes 1984, *Meditations on First Philosophy*, p. 189.

10. *Ibid.*, p.195.

11. See Deigh 1993.

12. See Damasio 1994, Greenspan 1988, Meyers 1997, and Kleinman and Good 1985. See also Glick and Bone 1990.

13. This is the kind of dual attention that anthropologists immersed in other people's worlds strive for and has been labeled the stance of the "participant–observer." Recent anthropologists critically evaluate this stance; for example, see Kleinman 1995. Interestingly, Aring seems to have something like this in mind when he urges physicians to have a "double awareness."

14. See Greenspan, p. 87.

15. For further reading along these lines, see Mills and Kleinman 1988.

16. Just because a spontaneous emotion is hard to change does not mean that it is determined biologically. For example, a person with a certain upbringing might automatically feel guilt in certain situations. In the next section, I discuss emotional attitudes such as homophobia that are inflexible for psychological reasons.

17. De Sousa argues that emotions play a critical role in "determining salience" for embodied human beings. De Sousa 1987.

18. Basch 1983.Note that Basch takes resonance emotions at birth to be examples of "fixed action patterns," which are reflex arcs that involve cortical functioning.

19. Tomkins 1963.

20. De Sousa 1987.

21. An important philosopher who argued for the value of resonance was David Hume. Hume uses the term "sympathy" to refer to spontaneous emotional resonance. Interestingly, one of the passages in which he describes sympathy explicitly refers to the problems of resonating in a medical context: "We may begin with considering a-new the nature and force of sympathy. The minds of all men are similar in their feelings and operations, nor can any one be actuated by any affection, of which all others are not, in some degree, susceptible. As in strings equally wound up, the motion of one communicates itself to the rest; so all the affections readily pass from one person to another, and beget correspondent movements in every human creature. . . .Were I present at any of the more terrible operations of surgery, 'tis certain, that even before it begun, the preparation of the instruments, the laying of the bandages in order, the heating of the irons, with all the signs of anxiety and concern in the patient and assistants, wou'd have a great effect upon my mind, and excite the strongest sentiments of pity and terror." Hume 1978 (1740).

22. It would be a mistake to imply that there is some "average" duration or developmental norm in which feelings should be processed. Given the diversity of human attachments and tragedies, such a standard would be ridiculous. However, it may be that with certain important exceptions, such as severe grief, a normative standard exists of ebbing and flowing, so that even strong emotions do not dominate one's attention so completely that one cannot be influenced emotionally by new experiences.

23. Segal et al. 1996.

24. The doctor does not hold two contradictory *beliefs*, since she has no negative

beliefs about homosexuals. Rather, the inconsistency is that her affects are not appropriate to her cognition

25. The distinction between holding an emotional point of view and holding a belief is a central point made by Cheshire Calhoun. See Calhoun 1984.

26. Of course, a huge moral as well as psychological difference exists between disgust on seeing blood and disgust at homosexuality, precisely because the latter involves interpreting another's ways of living and loving as disgusting.

27. See Beck 1979.

28. See Barlow 1988.

29. Although such errors cannot be avoided simply by detaching, cutting-edge medical school curricula are helping medical students recognize typical cognitive errors that are made in emotionally stressful situations. For example, physicians can learn to notice errors in how they "frame" medical dilemmas. Recall, for example, that physicians tend to overtreat patients subject to iatrogenic harm. See Kahneman and Tversky 1982.

30. Yager et al. 1984.

31. We commonly assume that only that that can be observed is real, that physical objects, spoken words, and other external events are the building blocks of reality. Social facts of experience are typically considered valid only insofar as they are tied to discrete observable facts.

32. Yet moods do seem to have shared developmental origins. For example, grieving involves feeling vulnerable or weakened, because nothing one can do can bring about the missed person's return. These feelings seem, on the face of them, to relate to a dependent infant's need for a caretaker who is not immediately available, given that an infant has no sense of time and therefore might be presumed to feel yearning or loss rather than simply impatience. However, we need to be very careful to avoid unsubstantiated empirical claims here. For people (children or adults, but not infants) with language, we know that yearning is a complex admixture of desire and despair. Attributing *this* emotion to an infant involves already seeing the infant in a complex psychological and social state, and not merely responding with simple resonance to a typical external situation.

33. Bowlby 1982 and Kübler-Ross 1975.

34. From a consultation with a physician discussed in Stein, 1985.

35. Wollheim 199, p. 15.

36. Lipsyte 1998.

37. For example, in a depressed mood "one expects failure and punishment." See Hirschfeld and Shea 1995 and Deckard et al. 1994.

38. Certainly, they do owe it to their patients to get help if they become clinically depressed or suffer from anxiety, mania, or other symptoms that impact their concentration. Programs are being developed to help physicians understand their own personal vulnerabilities as well as the more general risks of burn-out associated with adopting "uncaring" approaches to patients. See Deckard et al. 1994.

39. Lester et al. 1995.

40. For example, the standard of care in psychiatry is shifting from prescribing medication only for severe depression toward considering medication if a patient is not getting as much out of life as she *should*. Of course, this may be a response to aggressive marketing by both pharmaceutical and managed care corporations, as alleged in recent periodicals. See Cottle 1999.

41. Baxter 1992.

42. Iincreasingly effective biological treatments are being developed for emotional disorders. However, there are also powerful treatments for cognitive, or "thought," disorders. In fact, cognitive and affective disorders are usually intertwined in their presenting symptoms as well as in their treatments. For example, a person whose eating disorder manifests as a cognitively unrealistic body image and another with an eating disorder that presents primarily as depression may respond similarly to medication. So the existence of biologic remedies does not prove that emotions are merely biologically determined, reason-resistant events any more than it proves the same about thoughts. Other evidence used to argue for reductionist explanations of emotions includes data showing that stimulating certain neurons causes repetition of characteristic emotional experiences. However, neuroscientists such as Antonio Damasio argue that most likely there are neuronal pathways that we will be able to identify corresponding to higher thought processes, including the most rational, autonomous act of reason. However, knowing the mechanism does not explain the intentional content of the thoughts and therefore should not be assumed to provide an explanation of the meaning content of the emotions. Rather than invoke biologic reductionism to explain emotions, one can acknowledge the biologic basis of all human events and yet still look at how social, psychological, and biologic events interact. See Damasio 1994.

43. Seligman 1991.

44. However, there are some aspects of the cognitive reframing that Seligman suggests that could interfere with professional responsibility. He describes how people can free themselves from depressing self-blame by viewing unfortunate events as the result of transient impersonal circumstances rather than of their own character or limitations. This de-emphasis on personal responsibility, then, is at odds with the way physicians are trained to take a great deal of responsibility for the processes and outcomes of health care. I am indebted to Richard Myers for pointing out this conflict.

45. Joseph Fell argues that this dichotomy between emotions as self-soothing but ineffective versus detached reason as practical and effective is a pervasive one in the work of Jean-Paul Sartre. See Fell 1965.

46. Sartre 1975 (1948). See also Solomon 1984.

47. Sartre's view represents the strong claim that emotions are self-deceiving. Because of his complex view of the self, or subject, his view cannot be narrowly reduced to the claim that emotions seek to preserve "self-esteem." That is, he does not think there is a preexisting continuous "self," but rather that we are always engaged in a project of self-creation.

48. Philosopher Ronald De Sousa also describes emotions as involving "bootstrapping," in which people attribute to external situations features that correspond to their own emotional point of view. Yet he distinguishes instances of emotions that are amenable to realistic input and correction from those in which the emotion insulates a person from reality. The latter are more like the exceptional concretized states I discuss in chapters 1 and 6. De Sousa 1987, pp. 236–244.

49. Sartre could argue, as do economists who believe in rational self-interests, that in some complex way interests in others are still serving egoistic needs. Yet this would still be compatible with emotions seeking social success, and therefore, by my argument, a certain kind of realism.

50. According to the Kantian and Cartesian traditions, a dichotomy exists between theoretical and practical reason. Practical reasoning guides us in the world but does not

fundamentally reveal truth. It is only the detached position of the theoretical knower that provides sufficient "openness" to see things as they really are. Although I reject these views for knowledge of human emotional experience, I leave open the possibility that there could be disinterested knowledge, such as in theoretical mathematics, that does not answer to any human interest except an interest in truth.

51. Recently, philosophers ranging from Wittgenstein in the analytic tradition to Heidegger in the phenomenologic tradition have rejected the idea that reality is best apprehended from a practically disengaged point of view. These thinkers make the common point that, as human beings, we are in the world in a fundamentally interested way. They argue that we come to know the world by living in it, not by forming a picture of it in our heads. See Wittgenstein 1958 and Heidegger 1962 and 1977.

52. See O'Shaughnessy 1980.

53. What is interesting about this example is that something as practical as knowing how to move one's body had been automatically rejected as genuine knowledge of reality by Descartes and rationalist thinkers because such knowledge does not originate in detached reason. Descartes emphasizes the deceptiveness of body sense in his example of phantom limb pain, in *Meditations on First Philosophy*, p. 179.

54. It may be that a certain amount of idealization is an important part of physicians' functioning in caring for people facing suffering, death, and dying. For example, one physician described his own emotional struggle in caring for a cancer patient who refused medical treatment and was angry at his doctors. As Dr. Linnett came to empathize with this man's reasons for refusing treatment, he not only felt a sense of understanding and regard for the patient as a complex person, but idealized him. Linnett writes "I learned more from him about cancer than from any textbook." Linnett 1988.

55. A study of physicians in managed care stated that of those who considered themselves under great organizational pressures, "35% reported high levels of depersonalization in their patient interactions." See Deckard et al. 1994. In its most dramatic form, depersonalization (as well as an attachment to eugenic ideals) was used by doctors during the Nazi regime to maintain a sense of themselves as good people. Yet they perpetuated enormous cruelty and performed inhuman killings. See Lifton, 1986. I am not comparing the horrific actions of Nazi doctors to occupational burn-out of physicians in bureaucracies. Rather, the two situations, though highly distinct, illustrate how emotional adaptation can come at the cost of realism and sensitivity. All of this underlines the need for doctors to look beyond relationships with individual patients to broader social forces. To preserve their sense of integrity, physicians should develop professional standards and processes of accountability.

56. Aristotle says of emotions, "To feel them at the right time, with reference to the right objects, towards the right people, with the right motive, and in the right way, is what is both intermediate and best, and this is characteristic of virtue." Section 6, 1106b, in Aristotle 1988. See also Book II, Section 5, 1105b. I am grateful to Mariah Merritt for emphasizing Aristotle's relevance here. See also Kosman 1980.

57. A study of five distinct approaches that physicians take to patient relationships demonstrated that physician satisfaction was lowest in the narrowly biomedical and highest in the psychosocial (emotional communication) approach. See Roter et al. 1997.

FOUR

The Concept of Clinical Empathy

This book is inspired in part by a growing body of research showing that emotional communication in the patient–physician relationship positively influences healing.[1] Coinciding with this, medical school curricula and professional codes now emphasize training physicians to develop empathy.[2] However, widespread confusion exists over what constitutes empathy and how to achieve it. Empathy has been described in a variety of ways, such as "an end result, a tool, a skill, a kind of communication, a listening stance, a type of introspection, a capacity, a power, a form of perception or observation, a disposition, an activity, or a feeling."[3] Current theories of empathy do little to clarify the confusion, because, as this chapter argues, they overlook the possibility of a cognitive benefit from emotional engagement and therefore have no concept of emotional reasoning. That is, these views can be understood as falling into the two traditions of the patient–physician relationship outlined in chapter 1: those that emphasize detached knowledge and those that emphasize sympathy.

Ms. G.'s doctors showed how limited these two approaches are. The medical team, the ethicist, and the supervising psychiatrist adhered to the detachment norm, being careful not to let feelings of sympathy, pity, or their desire to rescue Ms. G. interfere with their objective decision-making process. On the other hand, Ms. G.'s internist sympathized with Ms. G., and in so doing seemed to identify too closely with her despairing view of her future. In both cases, the doctors clearly believed they were adhering to the norms of the medical profession.

In this chapter, I argue that neither detached cognition nor sympathetic merging lead to an experiential understanding of another person's distinct emotional perspective, the goal of empathy. In rejecting these approaches, I develop an alternative model of empathy based on emotional reasoning. Examining the constraints of the earlier theories allows emotions to emerge in a new role—as guides to another person's emotional perspective.

Clinical Empathy as Detached Insight

First, let us return to our discussion of Aring, Blumgart, and Osler's picture of clinical empathy as detached insight to see how this view falls short. These authors attempt to distinguish empathy, as an intellectualized stance, from the ordinary sympathy that doctors such as Hooker relied on. They presume that rather than being subject to sympathy, a physician can observe a patient's emotional life and use his knowledge of other people's emotional reactions (Blumgart and Osler) or of his own previous experiences (Aring) to make inferences about the patient's feelings.[4]

Blumgart and Osler seem to presuppose that knowing *how* a patient feels is no different from knowing *that* a patient is in a certain emotional state. When used to refer to third-person or impersonal knowledge about a state of affairs, such as the workings of bodies, the term *knowing how* is interchangeable with the term *knowing that*. Knowing *how* the stomach puts out gastric acid is a matter of knowing *that* histamine cells stimulate the release of certain hormones. Accordingly, knowing *how* a patient feels involves making correct inferences about her state, such as knowing *that*, as a matter of fact, she is sad instead of anxious.

Osler, for example, emphasizes that the physician's capacity to neutralize his emotions allows him to "see into" and hence "study" the patient's "inner life."[5] This claim presupposes that the physician can "project" before his "mind's eye" the patient's "inner life" as if it were "an image, as from a transparent slide, upon a screen."[6] Osler also assumes that the physician can "see into" his own "inner life" in order to recognize what he has in common with the patient. This use of visual metaphors underscores the stance of detachment, because a viewer stands apart from what he observes.

Although Osler mentions the physician's awareness of his own inner life, he does not give this awareness a cognitive role in understanding the patient's emotions. Aring, on the other hand, describes the use of introspection to better understand how the patient might feel. However, Aring's account of the relationship between emotions and cognition is not fundamentally different from Osler's. He, too, presumes that detached cognition does all the work of empathy. Aring, Blumgart, and Osler represent different versions of a common account of empathy as bifurcated into distinct cognitive steps. First, a physician accrues emotional wisdom, whether through observing other patients, or through introspection and, second, this already conceptualized emotional knowledge is used to infer, in a logical fashion, the facts about a patient's emotional state.

This account of empathy as inference does not explain how the communication between patient and physician can produce meanings that transcend the doctor's pre-existing concepts about emotions. To illustrate how the detached insight model cannot lead to empathic understanding, we can consider its two variations: drawing cognitive inferences after observing a patient's expressions and other behaviors or, as Aring advocated, including introspection in the process. First, consider whether observing others could be sufficient for empathy. While careful observation of another's words and gestures certainly contributes to empathic understanding, the object of empathy is not another's observable behavior—her words, gestures, and so on—but, rather, what is salient from her interior perspective.

Accordingly, the aim of empathy is not to label a patient's emotional state; empathy is needed even when it is quite obvious what emotional label applies to a patient. For example, a physician may observe that a patient is visibly angry and think that this observation alone gives him an understanding of the patient's emotional perspective. But it does not, just as Ms. G.'s doctors' awareness of her despair did not allow them fully to understand the concretized beliefs involved in her conviction that she had a hopeless future. Empathy requires attention to how a patient feels about specific issues. This sort of attention has great clinical relevance. For example, a cancer patient may be angry because she feels that her doctor, although a so-called expert, has made some superficial errors that signify to her that he may be making more serious errors and not treating her disease properly. While she might express superficial irritation at his carelessness (for example, forgetting some relatively insignificant aspect of her past medical history), she might feel deep anger at the thought that he might be careless about a serious aspect of her treatment. It is this emotional view of him as a serious threat, not her irritation at his mistake, that needs to be addressed.[7]

To fail to make such discriminations would, in this example, be to think that the patient is furious about the superficial error, an assumption that could lead the doctor to resent the patient rather than to respect her concern. Likewise, merely labeling the patient's feeling could also cause the doctor to sympathize with the patient's anger without really understanding it, and doing that could make the patient feel patronized. In contrast, the physician who can see the fear of negligent cancer treatment behind the patient's apparently overly angry reaction at a minor incident will be more effective. The understanding involved in clinical empathy is not observing that, as a matter of fact, a patient is in an emotional state, but noticing what is salient for the patient from within her emotional perspective.

This first, simple point already seriously undermines the cognitive insight model of empathy. If the physician relies strictly on detached observation and previous generalizations about affective experience, she will serve the patient poorly. She will miss important features of the patient's individual experience that are not contained in her generalizations, and she will expect typical reactions that may not occur in this patient. Even if a doctor gathers a great deal of factual information in a sincere effort to understand the patient's psychology, something important will be missing. The clinician would be like someone who goes to the theater but only notices those aspects of the drama that are described in the written program synopsis. She would not feel the sadness, frustration, or joy of the characters, but rather would observe that the characters were sad, frustrated, or joyful. In a clinical situation, a physician who knows that a patient fears her cancer has recurred but does not hear her specific concerns, may not know how to alleviate her anxiety. If the doctor's comments are too generic the patient may not develop the trust needed to reveal her history, thus hindering a therapeutic alliance.[8]

Even Aring's variation on the detachment model, in which the physician's own emotions play a role, fails to address this problem. Aring recognizes the limits of merely observing a patient's behavior and therefore describes the physician as introspecting—looking into his own mind and recalling his past experiences—in order to gain a more subtle understanding of the patient's emotions.

Yet despite this moment of introspection, Aring still locates empathy in the intellect of the physician rather than in emotional communication between patient and physician. In fairness to Aring, a physician who worked with him described him as a caring, effective physician. Perhaps he had a wider range of mental processes in mind than the term "introspection" suggests.[9] However, his written recommendations represent a version of the detached insight model of empathy, which claims that a physician can detachedly observe the patient and correctly apply knowledge of emotions derived from previous introspection.

What Aring's model presumes is that doctors can use cognitive concepts to pick out, from their own storehouse of accrued emotional knowledge, the themes that they detect patients are feeling. One error in this model is that the term *introspection*, which seems to describe a mechanism for direct self-knowledge, is actually a metaphor for a complex, socially mediated process.

According to the philosopher Ernst Tugendhat in his writings on knowledge of self and other, the whole idea of direct introspective knowledge of ourselves is a myth, because our own motives are not something of which we have direct knowledge. Tugendhat rejects the very idea on which Aring depends—that we can find a secure basis for knowledge of our own thinking in the insight we have of our thought processes. He sees self-knowledge as requiring a third-person view of our own behavior, meaning that we need to observe ourselves at the same time we feel our feelings to come to know our motives. From this he argues that we can attribute motives to ourselves in social relations reliably only in the way we attribute such motives to others—by considering our own actions, retrospectively, as they fit into relevant patterns.[10] When the term *introspection* is used to mean awareness of one's own complex emotional attitudes, it cannot be understood to refer to a mental act of direct intuition, the internal equivalent to external sense perception. Rather, the term *introspection* is a metaphor for a complex set of activities, including imagining, recollecting, and observing one's past emotions and social behaviors.

The model of empathy based on introspection and inference is, therefore, faulty and does not explain how a physician can detach herself emotionally and yet "see into" her own mind to produce concepts relevant to the patient's experience. We do not find a trustworthy source of direct emotional knowledge in introspection and cannot base empathy on intro-spection. We come to understand ourselves, as we come to know other people, through living in a world of social meanings, and we depend on these meanings to make sense of ourselves, even in our interiority.

The larger claim that Osler, Aring, and Blumgart make is that empa-thy is a form of theoretical reasoning rather than a form of experiential knowledge. Even knowledge gained by introspection, according to Aring, is transformed into concepts and applied to the patient's case. By this method, a physician applies conceptual knowledge to theorize what a patient's emotional condition is about. For example, observing a patient's prolonged silence and downward gaze would be grounds for generating competing hypotheses about the patient's mood, around which further data could be gathered. Once a decision was arrived at, a new set of questions could follow, without the physician ever leaving a theoretical standpoint.

My central claim is that empathy requires experiential, not just theo-retical, knowing. The physician experiences emotional shifts while listen-ing to the patient. The difference between knowing about something and experiencing something can be illustrated by taking a detour. Consider the two very different attitudes a person can take toward an action. One can take either the attitude of an experiencing agent or the attitude of an ob-server. An agent can have direct knowledge that he intends to perform an action, whereas an observer can only speculate that a person may perform an act. For example, a person *intends* to stand up, and therefore has a special grasp of the fact that standing is about to occur. He knows that standing is about to happen in the sense that events are organized in his field of inter-est around standing up. In contrast, an observer can only predict that stand-ing may occur, based on inferences from prior events and theory. Now, the difference between the observer and the agent is not that the agent is right more often. It may be that the agent intends to lift a thousand pounds, and the observer finds this extremely unlikely, so that the observer is more likely to be right than is the agent about the lifting. The point is that the observer can *only* make predictions about the agent, but the agent does not need to make third-person predictions to anticipate her own acts. She can antici-pate her acts directly, in the first-person, through forming intentions that lead to striving and, when physically possible, successful action.

The version of empathy as detached inference likens the empathizer to an observer, whose only way of anticipating the other's emotions is through prediction. A stance of prediction involves remaining equidistant from various possibilities in a field of unrealized possibilities. If the empathizing physician were like a detached observer rather than a participant, she could simultaneously entertain the possibility that the patient's gaze expresses sadness and the idea that the patient is engrossed in stimulating thoughts. This hypothetical stance would lend itself to scientific inquiry—one could apply earlier social science research and estimate the likelihood that people expressing themselves in this way are feeling one emotion or another. However accurately human emotions can be identified in this way (research has been done on reading facial expressions, for example), this form of hypothesizing and data gathering does not yield an understanding of the particular terrain of an individual's emotional state of mind. Again, the content of empathy—the features of emotional experience from a first-person perspective—sets constraints on the mode of reasoning proper to empathy. Applying concepts and making predictions constitute an inadequate mode for gaining a first-person sense of emotional experience. Empathic understanding is more like the first-person experiential knowledge of an agent anticipating her own acts than it is like the third-person predictions of an observer. It is not a theoretical or hypothetical standpoint, but an experiential stance.[11]

This is not to say that empathy identifies only one emotional state and cannot apprehend complex, or mixed, emotions. A physician can empathize with a patient who is ambivalent. For example, an adult child providing home care for a father with advanced Alzheimer's disease might express both sadness and relief on learning that her father has severe pneumonia and may die. A physician can empathize with this complex mix of feelings. Yet this differs from estimating that the adult child *might* be sad and that she *might* be relieved and making predictions accordingly.

Although empathy is not about making predictions, it does resemble hypothesizing in one way. Empathy involves learning from trial and error, or, more precisely, accurate empathy depends upon a physician's openness to ongoing feedback and correction. However, the need for feedback, or learning by trial and error, characterizes many forms of experiential knowledge that do not involve truly generating hypotheses or making predictions. Consider the practical knowledge involved in knowing how to dance—one learns to dance by practicing and making mistakes. Yet it is clear that knowing how to dance is not a matter of testing hypotheses. A dancer whose knowledge was based on predicting where her feet might go next would certainly be a sight to see!

The dance analogy, which will be evoked again later in the chapter, should not be taken too literally, however. Although empathy involves knowing *how*, not just knowing *that*, it is not reducible to knowing how to *do* something, like knowing how to dance. Knowledge about another's emotions, is not reducible to knowing how to behave in the presence of another's emotions, for example, to demonstrate listening. Rather, the knowing involved in empathy involves perceiving and imagining and is, therefore, cognitive as well as practical.

In summary, empathy is an experiential way of knowing about another's emotional states. We can say, then, that it impoverishes the concept of clinical empathy to reduce it to something like weather forecasting, in which one predicts the other's emotional conditions. Rather, the empathizer must be sufficiently affected by the patient's "weather" to be able to recognize and appreciate, in some quasi-first-person way, how the rain and sun feel. Sawyier, a philosopher of science, notes that "when we fill in the concept of empathy, part of what we imply is that the empathizer has himself had something happen to him right then; it is not just that he has thought hard, or tried to figure something out."[12] The detached insight model is insufficient because it denies the two experiential poles of empathic understanding: the empathizer grasps, more or less, how another person experiences her situation and at the same time experiences the other's attitudes as presences, rather than as mere possibilities.[13]

Aesthetics and the Origins of the Concept of Empathy

The detached insight model does not allow the possibility that discerning another's emotional state of mind is more like aesthetic or moral perception than like detached reasoning. That is, aesthetic and moral features of experience are not so clearly demarcated that one can apply predetermined concepts sufficiently to appreciate what is at stake. Rather, discerning that a situation has certain aesthetic or moral features in the first place—for example, noticing that a landscape is beautiful or that, of all human needs, a particular one exerts a special moral pressure—is a critical aspect of aesthetic or moral judgment.[14] Similarly, empathy is about noticing what is salient from another person's emotional perspective.

Leaving behind the detached insight model permits us to explore another model of empathy that comes from the field of aesthetics, in particular the German theorist Theodor Lipps. In 1903, Lipps defined empathy, or *Einfühlung*, as "the power of projecting one's personality into (and so fully comprehending) the object of contemplation," the same definition used today by the *Oxford English Dictionary*.[15] The metaphorical nature of this definition suggests that some of the confusion over the nature of *clinical* empathy derives from the ambiguity adhering to the general concept of empathy.

Lipps's model of the empathizer projecting his own personality into a passive object provides some important clues about how a form of cognition can be essentially affective. Lipps was primarily interested in understanding typical human gesture as depicted in art. His focus was on "expressive movements," which he defined as "movements of the body that manifest 'inner conditions.'"[16]

> *Einfühlung* is inherent in something perceived by me or in an element truly belonging to me and me only, i.e., something subjective, understood by me in the subject or in the spiritually corresponding object, but in the object for me or the object as it "looks" to the perceiving subject.

Lipps's emphasis here is on the essentially experiential nature of *Einfühlung*. By "subjective" he means "experiential," where experience has the sense of *Erlebnis*, or lived, first-hand experience. *Einfühlung* literally means "feeling into," by which Lipps has in mind a mode of perception that is essentially affective. *Einfühlung* is characterized by the essential connection between the affective feelings of the empathizer and the perceptual object of empathy. For Lipps, therefore, the phrase "projecting one's personality" refers most generally to the *experience* of a connection between one's own affective condition and the object one is trying to understand.

In the kind of *Einfühlung* directed toward understanding a living person, Lipps notes, the gestures and expressions of that person

> are not the "man," they are not the strange personality with his psychological equipment, his ideas, his feelings, his will, etc. All the same, to us, the man is linked to these manifestations. The imaginative, feeling, willing, individual is immediately apparent to us through his sensuous appearances, i.e., his manifestations of life. In a movement, grief, spite, etc., is perhaps apparent to us. This connection is created through *Einfühlung*.[17]

Here Lipps argues that the emotions of another living person are not apparent to us except insofar as we pre-reflectively, or automatically, project our own emotions into him, just as we do when we imbue an inert object, such as a work of art, with meaning. The empathizer must reach beyond what is apparent to grasp, through physical movements, the psychological life of another person.

At the heart of these accounts is a claim that stands in opposition to the prevalent detached insight model in medicine, the claim that grasping another's emotions involves having an experience. Yet, perhaps because Lipps is interested primarily in appreciating works of art, he does not link empathy with an interpersonal exchange. While useful, then, the concept of *Einfühlung* is insufficient to account for *clinical* empathy.

Lipps's model of empathy is important, however, because it contributes the controversial idea that empathy differs from detached cognition insofar as the observer's own emotions organize and direct her understanding. This idea of emotions directing attention was prevalent in thinkers from diverse fields in the late nineteenth and early twentieth century and is most systematically argued for by Martin Heidegger, whose philosophical views were already mentioned in chapter 2. Though he does not address the question of empathy in particular, Heidegger argues that general human knowledge of reality is guided by having shared affective possibilities. He argues that it is by having, or being in, "moods" that we organize activities with shared social meanings, whether these activities are as basic as building things and procuring food or as complex as dealing with foreknowledge of our mortality and finding existential life projects.[18] For Heidegger, what makes it possible to *understand* something is the prior possibility of being in relation to that thing, where *being* means existing—including the full range of affective and volitional activities.

It is in this sense that empathy presupposes a common human set of interests and moods. The point is not just that the empathizer must be in some mood or other, for this is true of all being-in-the-world (Heidegger's term).[19] The empathizer must be in a mood that is interested in the human predicament that another faces. The philosopher Edmund Husserl (who was Heidegger's teacher) said that in empathy, one person regards the other as "an-other" self, that is, as another center of an emotional world.[20]

However, two points need clarification in applying Heidegger and Husserl's philosophic abstractions to the phenomenon of clinical empathy. First, it is critical to note that their emphasis is on common human *possibilities*, rather than on people actually sharing similar experiential histories. Two people with distinct actual histories still share possibilities. A non-grieving physician who is nevertheless motivated by attachments and vulnerable to loss will attend to the nuances of a patient's grief, including the impact the grief has on the patient and how she tolerates it, in part because of their common human vulnerabilities.

A second caveat, then, in applying Heidegger's ideas is that he is not speaking of human interests in a narrow psychological sense. To see in others only what is relevant to one's own self-interest, that is, to one's particular needs or wishes, would be extremely stifling and isolating; one could never learn anything new about others if one referenced all of their experiences in terms of one's direct concerns. Rather, the empathizer can be interested even when another's feelings represent foreign concerns to her. She can imagine those concerns because of her interest in common human struggles and emotions. It is precisely in such cases that empathy shows its power to bridge differences.[21] We are fundamentally interested in a broader range of human experiences than those that serve our narrow self-interests. This sense in which empathy can be both "interested" and "disinterested" relates to the possibility of being emotionally responsive without over-identifying, or projecting one's own narrow interests onto another.

By using Heidegger to draw out the implications of Lipps's discussion of *Einfühlung*, then, we can discard the vague phrase "projection of one's personality" and characterize empathy in the following way: an essentially experiential understanding of another person that involves an active, yet not necessarily voluntary, creation of an *interpretive* context. Heidegger's focus on shared possibilities, rather than actualities, is, in my view, essential for emphasizing how physicians, who in no way share patients' actual predicaments, may share a range of imagined possibilities. What is critical, however, is that what physicians imagine be relevant to patients' actual experiences. How does this occur?

Psychoanalytic Views of Empathy as Affective Merging

In the clinical setting, the question of how a physician can be guided to imagine a patient's distinct situation accurately has, to my knowledge, yet to be addressed. There has been a sustained attempt by psychoanalysts to describe empathy, but Heidegger's distinction between sharing affective possibilities and actually being in the same, real mood has been missed. Lipps's unfortunate phrase—"projection of one's personality"—is read as meaning projecting oneself into another, implying a merging of persons. Those psychoanalysts and psychologists who equate empathy with a merging identification between patient and therapist take this implication further. I turn to their views next in order to lay the groundwork for a model of empathy that, while interpersonal, does not involve merging.

The psychoanalytic discourse on empathy, with roots in Freud, Deutsch, Fliess, and Fenichel, and given seminal formulation by Heinz Kohut, emphasizes the clinician's capacity to coexperience emotions with the patient. Though each of their views is complex, they share several key assumptions, which I consider here. In 1926, Helene Deutsch hypothesized that empathy involves an unconscious identification between therapist and patient in which the therapist feels the patient's experiences to be her own, and recognizes only on reflection that the source of the feelings is the patient.[22] Fliess, in 1942, described the therapist regressing to a state in which his ego boundaries are weakened and he can experience the patient's inner state from within himself.[23] And in 1953, Fenichel wrote about the therapist's "narcissistic identification" with the patient, which involves the "taking over by the subject of the object's inner state."[24] Most recently and influentially, Kohut equated empathic feeling with bracketing from consciousness the distinction between self and other. In a 1959 essay, he posited that one can refrain from critical thinking in order to experience an unbounded continuum between another's feelings and one's own. The therapist's capacity to feel what the patient feels allows her to identify with the patient to the degree that she can temporarily experience a sense of herself and the patient as one person, thereby gaining access to how it feels to be in the patient's concrete situation.[25]

These descriptions of merging are metaphorical, as indeed are all descriptions of empathy.[26] To consider their accuracy, we need to seek greater precision and ask if these analysts provide an account of how, by sharing an affect, one attains accurate empathic understanding. My reading is that the mechanism they hold in common involves taking emotional resonance to be a way of directly sampling what a patient's emotional state of mind is like.

This account is an important corrective to the model of detached insight because of its emphasis on direct emotional attunement. My argument against it is that, although resonance does contribute to empathy, it is not sufficient for grasping another's distinct emotional perspective. Recall from the last chapter that resonance is spontaneous affect that is similar to another's affect, such as feeling anxious around an anxious person or instantly light-hearted in the presence of a joyful person. Almost every psychoanalytic account of empathy, from Freud on, assigns some role to resonance, described as the therapist finding herself feeling "automatically" sad or happy with the patient without relying on any effort of thought. [27] I do not disagree with the clinical observation that resonance and empathy are closely related, but question the theoretical claim that resonance itself yields empathic understanding.

At a practical level, the problem is how to relate the fact of resonance to the cognitive tasks involved in empathy. It seems to me essential to distinguish *individual* events of resonance from the complex understanding involved in empathy. Consider, for example, a commonplace experience in which one person responds to another person's tears with "automatic" tears or to her laughter with spontaneous laughter. Despite the shared affect, one person may have no sense of what the other is crying or laughing about.[28,29]

Insofar as resonance involves little cognitive content of its own, it is insufficient for grasping another's distinct emotional point of view. Recall that recognizing that a patient is angry is insufficient for achieving empathy. Rather, empathy seeks to discern what, specifically, the patient feels angry about. If the physician simply resonates with a patient who angrily points out a minor error that she has made, she might never address what the patient is really angry about. Emotional resonance is insufficient to instruct one about the particularities of another's emotional state.

Recall from chapter 3 the developmental theory that relates innate resonance to learning typical emotional meanings. Resonating in typical or common situations leads people to develop shared emotional meanings. The point of the developmental model, however, is to show that resonance occurring in the setting of a social, linguistic experience leads to the development of complex emotional content. Resonance does not, in and of itself, *generate* the shared content. Resonance is a precursor of more complex emotions that are learned through social experiences. Although, interestingly, simple resonance occurs later in life, particularly as a trigger to and component of empathic listening, the occurrence of objectless affect in adult life cannot do any more than it does in infancy. Resonance is like stage lighting or music in that it can attune people to common themes, but it cannot magically and silently present to those involved a common, complex emotional viewpoint.

Are there additional ideas about resonance that might make the merging model more coherent? Psychoanalysts who see resonance as sufficient for empathy presume that through feeling a common type of feeling, the therapist *identifies* with the patient's point of view. In relation to the role of resonance, Freud talks about the identification of the analyst with the analysand's *experiences*. His subtle point has been misconstrued to mean that through resonance, which is a shared "gut feeling," this identification is a direct happening or event, and the therapist or physician finds herself spontaneously sharing the patient's cognitively complex emotions.

However, no special psychoanalytic mechanism exists that could explain how resonance could yield an immediate grasp of a complex point of view. The strict psychoanalytic sense of *identification* refers to a phenomenon in which one person actually develops structural features of a personality as a result of imitating an admired (or feared) other. The most ubiquitous example of strict identification is the child's identification with a parent. For example, a boy repeatedly watches his father shave a certain way, and this becomes his lifelong pattern of shaving.[30]

Identification, in this sense, is a process that requires time and an in-depth connection with another person. Empathy in brief clinical encounters cannot consist of identification in this sense. It is a misunderstanding to equate identifying with a *person* with empathy, as Freud emphasized when he said that empathy does not involve identifying "with the other person per se, but with what he is experiencing."[31]

It is, in fact, dangerously wrong for a physician to presume that if she feels resonance, she immediately understands how a patient feels about her illness, her treatment, and her future. For example, consider this experience told to me by the patient. When this woman was pregnant she expressed fear of childbirth. Resonating with her anxiety, her obstetrician quickly reassured her that she could be kept from severe pain and that, if necessary, she could be medicated to the point that she would be "out of it." This response terrified her, because her fear was of losing control, either by being groggy from anesthesia or being "tied down" to an intravenous line. She had, it turns out, been a rape victim who had experienced this kind of helplessness and immobility.

Resonance is insufficient for achieving empathy. Another related problem with the merging model is that it presupposes that empathy involves bracketing from consciousness one's ordinary awareness of the distinction between self and other. However much Deutsch, Fliess, Fenichel, and Kohut emphasize that the therapist is ultimately responsible for maintaining awareness of the distinction between self and other, they see the mental act of empathy as fantasizing a merging of identities. Kohut, for example, claims that empathy involves two steps. First, in order to directly experience the patient's concrete feelings, one must set aside awareness of the distinction between oneself and the patient. Second, the clinician must reflectively distance herself from the patient to consider whether her experiential grasp of the patient fits with other data, including the patient's responses to her empathic communication.[32] The distinguishing characteristic of empathy, he argues, is that it involves fantasizing a "we" subject that unites oneself with another.

However, let us consider when, if ever, people can fantasize being part of a "we" subject. Moments that might be considered candidates for this occur during lovemaking or dancing, when two people seem to share one set of movements and feelings. The content of such moments is critically different from the content of clinical empathy, which is what it feels like to be in the patient's actual, individual life, feeling what she is feeling. That is, although (as I will argue) imagination and fantasy are involved in empathy, the content of empathy is the patient's individual experience and not a shared dyad of patient and physician undergoing a "we" experience.

A related argument against the merging model is that if what one is trying to do is imagine how another person feels, one never imagines this as oneself and the other being in the exact same situation. That is, during the experience of empathizing, or "feeling with" a patient, the physician always remains aware that she is not actually in the patient's situation. This point is well made by Edith Stein, a philosopher who, like Heidegger, was a student of Edmund Husserl in the early twentieth century. Stein offers a persuasive criticism of the claim that one must seemingly merge with another in order to understand what her feelings are like. Stein questions the claim that in the experiential moment of empathy, "there is no distinction between our own and the foreign 'I,' that they are one."[33]

In referring to the imagination, Stein argues that even at the moment of feeling with another, one does not take oneself to be in another's here-

and-now situation. Following Husserl, she argues that the sense of being "here and now" depends upon a sense of being in one's own body.[34] Stein compares empathy with recollection, given that both are *imaginative* experiences that "announce" the presence of a *real* "I" that is not actually "here and now." Thus, these experiences differ from pure fantasy, in which one creates an *unreal* subject. She describes recollection of a past experience as a detailed, imaginative reliving of the past. Recollection thus differs from mere recall in that in recollection, one re-experiences an imaginative connection to the past event, rather than simply positing that a certain event occurred that is causally related to one's present experience. But, Stein says, this filling-out experience of the past

> does not make the remembered experience primordial [here and now]. The present viewpoint of the remembered state of affairs is completely independent of the remembered viewpoint. I can remember a perception and now be convinced that I was formerly under a delusion. I remember my discomfort in an embarrassing situation and now think it was very funny. In this case the memory is no more incomplete than if I again take the former viewpoint.[35]

The same gap exists between the "I" who is the subject of the imaginative act of empathy and the "I" who is its object. She uses the example of a viewer watching an acrobat perform.[36] Stein points out that even if I am so absorbed in empathizing with the acrobat that I entirely forget myself and pick up a dropped program without even "knowing" I did so, I have not merged with the acrobat. For, if I reflect on the experience of dropping my program, it is apparent that this experience *was* given to me directly in the "here and now" (that is, sensed in my own body), even though that "here and now" is past and only given in memory. However, if I reflect on the acrobat's acts, it is apparent that the other's action was only announced, but never experienced directly in a past "here and now," an embodied moment, of mine. Stein says that empathy is an imaginative "announcement" and fulfilling explication of another "I," rather than an imagined merger forming a "we" subject.

Stein's analysis emphasizes the essential "as-if," or virtual, character of empathy, another aspect important to building a model for clinical empathy. We misspeak if we describe empathic absorption as a total immersion in, or merging with, another, because the inner quality of the act of empathy is never one of total merging.[37] That is, it is not just the *fact* that we must imagine what the other feels that makes empathy an *as-if*, rather than a directly given, experience. Even if one brackets the reflective awareness that one is not really in another's situation and considers only what seems to be happening within the imaginative world of empathy, one does not achieve a "merging" experience. It is the *internal* structure of empathy that requires an awareness that another's experiences are not actually present within my own sphere of experience. This relates to Husserl's contention that understanding a person as *another* person always includes an awareness of the *absence* of the other in one's own "primordial" situation; one cannot, for example, directly move the other's body or feel the other's physical pain.[38]

If we reject the view of empathy as involving even a fantasized merger between self and other, we have reason to seriously challenge the prevailing *Oxford English Dictionary* definition of empathy as "projecting one's personality into (and so fully comprehending) the object of contemplation." In their zeal to teach empathy, medical schools have unwittingly been deeply influenced by this inaccurate model. Medical students are taught to imagine *themselves* in their patients' shoes.

This differs from imagining what it is like to be in the patient's position. Note, however, that the ambiguity of the phrase blurs the distinction between self and other.[39] Empathy so defined is too easily confused with the psychological defense mechanism of projection. Projection is "the unconscious act or process of ascribing to others one's own ideas or impulses or emotions."[40] Several risks to medical care arise when physicians believe that empathy involves imbuing the patient's experience with their own sensibilities and preferences. These risks are illustrated by the already-mentioned case of the surgeon Christian Barnaard, who was driven to perform the first successful heart transplant operation. After the first transplant patient died, Barnaard felt so disappointed that he approached the next patient on his list, Philip Blaiberg, and spoke to this ill man as if they were both facing the same challenge. Jay Katz quotes Barnard as saying, "I feel like a pilot who has just crashed. . . . Now I want you, Dr. Blaiberg, to help me by taking up another plane as soon as possible to get back my confidence."[41] By merging Blaiberg's urgency with his own, Barnaard failed to attend to the difference between the experience of undergoing grueling, experimental surgery and enduring months in the intensive care unit, and that of being a surgeon needing to overcome a failure and pioneer a heroic treatment.

Barnaard lacked the capacity to *decenter*, or step aside from his own emotional perspective, and discern what distinct meanings the surgery had for Blaiberg. Decentering is as essential to clinical empathy as is resonance. Note that an important difference exists between decentering and detaching. Decentering involves imaginatively viewing a situation from the patient's position. This imagining is guided by a physician's own emotions, but the subject matter is not his own life. Empathy, then, is a much more complex activity than either the detached insight or the merging models describe. What these models fail to address is how a person can use his capacity to engage skillfully and emotionally with another in order to understand distinct aspects of the other person's experience. In the nursing profession, in which more attention had been paid to developing this skill, practitioners learn carefully to notice and regulate the use of their own emotions in assessing and communicating with patients. In discussing these skills, nurse–philosopher Patricia Benner emphasizes how skills like clinical empathy are cultural inventions quite distinct from the natural sympathy of people affiliating with each other. She observes how unnatural it is for health care providers to appreciate the emotional worlds of patients without confusing them with their own. She argues that the objectives of nursing, including alleviating pain and suffering, require carefully avoiding merging identifications with patients, even while striving for empathy.[42]

Psychiatrists, psychotherapists, and social workers also strive to develop their capacity to resonate emotionally with patients without becoming overly identified, projecting, or otherwise overreacting. Training in these fields emphasizes developing "boundaries," a term that focuses on distinctions between the role of the caregiver and the role of a friend. Although boundaries are often understood concretely as rules about external behaviors (e.g., therapists should not engage in business dealings with their patients), there is an assumption about emotional skills inherent to these rules. Therapists are expected to be flexible and open to understanding complex human experience, in part by decentering from their own narrow emotional reactions.

Clinical empathy, then, is related to Lipps's *Einfühlung* in its dependence on the empathizer's emotional participation, but it requires the empathizer to have a particular skill. The empathizer does not just happen to resonate; she cultivates the capacity for imagining perspectives to which she lacks immediate access. The challenge is to describe the precise way that resonance and awareness of the distinctness of another's situation contribute to this imagination work. I turn to this next.

A Model of Clinical Empathy as Emotional Reasoning

This chapter has laid the groundwork for a new account of clinical empathy that rejects the two common models of empathy—detached insight and affective merging—in favor of one in which the empathizer is able to resonate emotionally with, yet stay aware of, what is distinct about the patient's experience. It borrows from *Einfühlung* the idea of participating in another's experience but rejects the model of merging in favor of one in which the ability to resonate allows the curious physician to use her imagination. The imaginative use of the physician's affects provides a framework, or organizing context, for understanding the patient's particular experience.

The work fundamental to empathy is imagining *how* it feels to experience something, in contrast to imagining *that* something is the case. Two philosophers, Edward Casey and Richard Wollheim, describe the role of the imagination in understanding what an experience feels like. In the book *Imagining*, Casey describes imagining *how* as something more complex than mere "imaging," or imagining *that*:

> We are capable not only of imaging (objects and events) and imagining that (states of affairs obtain), but also of imagining how to do, think, or feel certain things, as well as how to move, behave, or speak in certain ways. There is a sense of personal agency, or the imaginer's own involvement in what is being imagined, which is lacking or at least muted in instances of sheer imagining-that. To imagine how is to project not merely a state of affairs *simpliciter* (i.e., one in which the imaginer is not a participant) but a state of affairs into which the imaginer has also projected himself (or a surrogate) as an active being who is experiencing how it is to do, feel, think, move etc., in a certain manner.[43,44]

In the case of empathy, imagining *how* is distinguished by the fact that the images and relations in the imagined world are organized from the perspective of an *agent*, rather than that of an external observer. For example, Casey says that in imagining how to lace up a boot, one would imagine the kinesthetic sensations involved in the action of bootlacing.[45]

The claim that imagining *how* is agent-centered applies to cases in which one imagines how two persons do something together, though it might seem that such cases do not require the viewpoint of an agent. Consider, for example, what happens when I imagine how person A gives person B a flower. If what I imagine could be described either from the perspective of the flower giver or the flower receiver, then the imaginative portrayal must itself be multivalent—it must be open to more than one perspective, rather than categorically organized from an agent's perspective. But, as Richard Wollheim points out, it is different to imagine how A gives B a flower than it is to imagine how B receives a flower from A. It may be possible to imagine both things, but only sequentially, never in one act. According to Wollheim, when one imagines how A experiences something, one "liberally and systematically intersperses imagining his doing certain things with imagining his feeling and thinking certain things."[46] I take Wollheim's point to be that in imagining how A feels, I follow the flow of A's feelings and thoughts as they would flow in life for an experiencing subject. If B's feelings are noticed, it is as they are read by A. For example, if I imagine B scowling at A, this scowl is felt as a rejection, its interpretation by A, rather than as whatever it felt like for B. If more "interior" awareness of B's feelings intervenes, then one is now imagining how it feels for B to receive flowers from A, and A will only be noticed as B would notice A.

How does this account of imagining *how* apply to the practice of clinical empathy? That is, does a doctor really have to use her imagination in this way to take a thorough history? Why is such a seemingly elaborate cognitive use of the emotions needed when reacting with automatic sympathy might be sufficient to communicate the doctor's concern to the patient? The best way for me to address this question is to relate a clinical experience from my own training that shows the distinction between automatic sympathy and selectively using resonance to imagine how the patient feels.

I was called to see Mr. Smith, who had been a successful executive, and a powerful figure in his family, when a sudden neurological disorder paralyzed him from the neck down, leaving him ventilator-dependent. His doctors and nurses were worried that he had suicidal intent because he would not communicate with them or participate in the physical therapy essential to his recovery. When I entered his room, I saw a helpless, locked-in, cathectic man, whose eyes showed a glimmer of interest in meeting the psychiatrist. I greeted him warmly, and, I later realized, sorrowfully. Gently, I asked him to talk with me. He struggled, trembling and red-faced, to speak a few words through his tracheostomy tube, then asked me to leave him to rest, and his eyes glazed over. I felt ashamed of having pushed him to make a futile effort.

I felt hopeless about returning to talk with him and thought that this reflected my own lack of clinical experience. However, another psychiatrist pointed out that my profound hopelessness about helping Mr. Smith likely reflected *his* own intense hopelessness. I was resonating with him, but attributing the feeling to my own difficulties as a physician. This helped me to decenter and become curious about how Mr. Smith felt about his situation.

I imagined what it would be like to be a powerful older man, suddenly enfeebled, handled by one young doctor after the next. I found myself moved to feel impatience, then rage at being trapped in a body that no one knew how to help. I felt mounting frustration and something else—a sense of shame. I reentered his room determined not to patronize or withdraw from him.

I looked him in the eyes and spoke in a robust voice more suited to a business interaction than to comforting someone who is hurt. I asked "What is it about talking with me that you don't like?" He did not look at me at first, but his manner shifted. He literally found his voice, whispering loudly through the tracheostomy that he was furious at the doctors for invading his privacy and exposing his family to so much. After all, he said, we were obviously too incompetent to figure out any way to help him.

I did not argue with him or exhort him to have hope. Rather, I stayed in the moment of anger with him, saying something about how infuriating it must be for a person of his strength to be paralyzed, trapped in the hospital, in front of his family. As I spoke he turned to look directly at me with tears in his eyes, and we began to work together.[47]

Although both empathy and sympathy involve emotional resonance, this case illustrates how empathy involves using resonance to attune to another's specific emotional views through imagination work. My initial sympathy was an unimaginative response to Mr. Smith's obvious vulnerability, which led me to treat him gently, as I would treat *any* injured person. In contrast, by imagining how he experienced his illness and disability, I was moved to an emotional sense of anger that became more complex, leading to a sense of underlying shame and helplessness. This case also highlights the practical importance of imagining how a particular upsetting situation feels versus simply recognizing that a patient is upset. I imagined being unable to move and feeling rage at being an object of pity before "my" family. Imagining these specific experiences guided my interactions with Mr. Smith, shaping the timing of my remarks and my body language to communicate my respect for him and my capacity to withstand his anger.

In empathy, emotional resonance can set the tone, but imagination work must be done to unify the details and nuances of the patient's life into an integrated affective experience. By "experience" I mean a sense of how it feels to have a certain illness, disability, or psychological injury. Of course, the physician's imagined experience may be an inaccurate representation of the patient's experience, and ongoing dialogue is necessary to develop accuracy.[48]

What gives empathic imagining the *quality* of reality or genuineness rather than that of simulation?[49] This is an especially problematic question because of the origins of the concept of *Einfühlung* in aesthetics, where the feelings that one empathizes with are already depicted in works of art, rather than present in another living person. Yet painters expressing moods, writers creating characters, and actors portraying roles seek to present emotions in an experiential way, from a first-person perspective. Dancers go one step further in that they use their own bodies to express another's emotions (or a choreographer's ideas about emotions). To explore the tension between genuineness and simulation in empathy, thinking about a dancer's use of emotions is particularly instructive, because it conjures up participatory rather than more intellectualized modes of portraying emotions.

The philosopher Susanne Langer describes the way a dancer portrays an emotion as a real holistic presence. Langer says: "The primary illusion of dance and the basic abstraction" is "virtual spontaneous gesture."[50] "Gesture," she reminds us, is defined as "expressive movement" and means two alternative things. "It means either 'self-expressive,' i.e., symptomatic of existing subjective conditions, or 'logically expressive,' i.e., symbolic of a concept, that may or may not refer to factually given conditions," she notes. She then explains that in dance, the dancer seems to be expressing her actual emotion, but she is, in fact, engaging in an imaginative act of embodying an emotion. She states that "the conception of a feeling disposes the dancer's body to symbolize it." She recognizes that it is very difficult to imagine the dancer taking on a feeling that is not her own. Yet this is possible, as illustrated by the example of a dancer in pain from a sore toe who embodies (and does not merely fake) joy in a dance. Also, she points out how sometimes a dancer emulates a mechanistic toy, taking on mechanistic type movements and embodying them as if her body were moved by the powers of such a mechanism. This, she believes, shows that the dancer can embody a variety of subjective states that will never genuinely be her own. That is, the dancer can direct her own kinesthetic sense to experience a rigidity and automaticity that differ from her usual way of comporting herself.

The joy the dancer expresses need not be *about* her own personal situation. "It takes precision of thought not to confuse an imagined feeling, or a precisely conceived emotion that is formulated in a perceptible symbol, with a feeling or emotion actually experienced in response to real events. Indeed, the very notion of feelings and emotions that are not really about us, but only about imagined experiences, is strange to most people."[51] She argues that one reason this is strange is that we tend to think of emotions as penetrating to the core of an individual, revealing the person's soul, so that it seems the dancer's feelings must be expressions of her individual soul. Langer claims that this assumption is incorrect. "If the person whose joys and pains the dance represents is none other than the dancer, the confusions between feeling shown and feeling represented, symptom and symbol, motif and created image, are just about inescapable."

The antidote to this, she argues, is to recognize how dancers *symbolize* affect in their gestures—they use bodily tensions and movements to embody affective states. This skill is, to her, fundamentally impersonal. When describing specific dances, writers "almost invariably speak of setting up tensions, exhibiting forces, creating gestures that *connote* feelings or even thoughts. The actual thoughts, memories, and sentiments that lie behind them are purely personal symbols that may help the artistic conception, but do not appear."

Langer's goal is to show that the dancer can portray a broader range of affect than arises from within her personal experience. Langer's view is relevant to this account of clinical empathy because, just as the dancer's movements are symbolic and not merely personal expressions, the physician's affect is not *about* the physician's own situation. It is significant that while imagining Mr. Smith's situation, I was able to say "he" or "I" interchangeably. As Casey points out, in imagining how an experience feels, the imagined subject can easily be left unspecified. For example, I did not have to see *myself* as personifying Mr. Smith to imagine *having* the experience he was undergoing.

The spontaneity of imaginative experience, whether in empathy or in dance, seems to rest on this power to landscape the scene with images from different people without having to explain their occurrence by the ordinary rules of empirical experience. Again, this quality of imagination points to the error in the "merging" model of empathy. The fact that empathy involves the physician's integration of her own affects and the patient's images does not entail that the physician must imagine *herself* in the patient's situation.[52] The examples above show that it is not necessary to specify that it is oneself in the imagined situation in order to imagine an experience from a participatory perspective.

The useful aspect of Langer's discussion for a model of empathy is her emphasis on how the dancer expresses emotions that are not her own by accessing a range of embodied expressions that humans hold in common. The idea is that dancers can be moved by emotions that neither originate in nor refer concretely to their own personal situations. I disagree with Langer's claim, however, that such participation is compatible with the dancer detaching from her own personal emotions. Langer's emphasis on how the dancer can express joy despite feeling preoccupied with her own sore toe is misleading in that she implies that the dancer has an emotion in her head that is independent of what she expresses through her body. In fact, I would argue that the dancer's skill lies not in her ability to detach, but in her ability to embody emotions at will. The special skill of the dancer is that she actually inhabits emotions that are not originally her own. She *participates* in joyful movements; she does not *imitate* them. This is what enables her authentically to express joy to others. She has a skilled relation to her body that frees her to express some things and not others, so that she can guide her body toward expressing joy even when her preexisting physical state is painful. The minute details of such skill may involve moving in ways that create less pain or in finding energy that makes her experience bodily joy. This skill—of genuinely moving oneself into alternative emotional, embodied states, as opposed to doing what comes naturally—makes the example of the dancer relevant to physicians, who need to be able to manage their pre-existing moods in order to pay empathic attention to patients.

Yet the dance analogy is insufficient for a model of clinical empathy for the following reason. It explains how physicians can attune themselves to patients insofar as patients provide clear choreography, or guidance, but it does not account for how, during empathy, new discoveries can be made by patient and physician together. Because I have emphasized that empathy is needed precisely because patients do not come to doctors with an already formulated sense of what troubles them, this is a serious limitation of this model.

This raises the question of how emotional attunement leads to discovering something new and specific about another's experience. In answering this question, what is still puzzling is that our models of cognition still treat learning something about another person and responding affectively as entirely distinct events. According to this view, all the cognitive work of empathy is done by detached reason, and emotional reactions simply follow each discovery.[53] In contrast, my claim is that experiencing emotion guides what one imagines about another's experience, and thus provides a direction and context for learning.

As the previous chapter on emotional reasoning showed, emotions are not necessarily pre-programmed and static, but, rather, involve making new linkages.[54] Here is where empathy depends upon specific properties of emotional reasoning—associative linking and moods that provide an organizing context. The development or movement of ideas in empathic understanding is essentially affective and experiential. In this sense, the thinking involved in empathy is more like the thinking involved in dreaming, in that one image is often connected to the next for emotional reasons. For example, fear or anger can motivate patterns of action in a dream, linking one thing to the next. Dreams cannot be divided into detached thoughts followed by emotional reactions; emotions *guide* the thoughts.[55]

Having an emotion can be integral to imagining something, as illustrated by Wollheim in the example of someone feeling erotic pleasure while having a sexual fantasy. His point is that erotic feelings organize the fantasy. In contrast, a person could have feelings that are reactions to having the fantasy, such as guilt feelings. Wollheim's point is that the fantasy experience could still be organized the same way without the guilt, but it could not be the same fantasy without the sexual feelings.

This helps clarify the view of empathy I have been building, beginning with Lipps's emphasis on participating in another's experience. I argued that this participation does not consist of affective merging. Rather than feeling what, specifically, another feels about a similar particular, I argued that the listener *imagines* how the experience feels. However, the kind of imagining involved in empathy is unified, or made coherent, through the same kind of linkages involved in dreaming or sexual fantasies. The movement from a more general to a more specific grasp of another person's feelings unfolds through a narrative that moves by emotional associations.

This also helps clarify the role of resonance in empathy. Resonance is extremely helpful for empathy because it provides a coordinated emotional context between speaker and listener. However, resonance does not always occur to trigger empathy, and the emotions that are stimulated by imagining how another feels are not, strictly speaking, instances of resonance. Recall that, by definition, resonance feelings lack focused cognitive content, whereas affective imagining in empathy has specific content. Whether empathy is triggered by resonance is not essential; what is needed is an emotional context for imagining another's situation. When supplied by spontaneous feeling, or resonance, the feelings are transformed as they are put to cognitive use. As the feelings take on complex cognitive focus or content, they become full-fledged emotional attitudes. So the use of resonance in the service of imagining another's emotional meanings transforms states of resonance into complex emotional dispositions that provide a context for the imagined experience.

Absent resonance, the process of imagining another person's experiences with a certain emotional openness can itself move one to take an emotional orientation or attitude that is attuned to another's state of mind. That is, as I imagine the particular meaning of another's grief, I can find myself in an emotional state that is not one I would otherwise be disposed to feel. In a context unrelated to empathy, Wollheim states "imagination can induce a particular emotional state in someone who does not have the emotional disposition that that state would ordinarily manifest."[56] In empathy, one experiences the imagined scenario affectively. That is why in the first part of this chapter, I emphasized that something happens to the empathizer: she is genuinely moved.

There are diverse pathways to empathy. Spontaneous resonance can be put to imaginative use, or lacking resonance, a physician may listen more carefully to a patient's story and find herself moved by the narrative. To become more reliable at empathizing with patients, physicians need to cultivate a way to trigger empathy when they do not spontaneously resonate with a patient. As I suggest in chapter 6 and the previous account of Mr. Smith, one way is to cultivate curiosity about what it feels like to be in the patient's distinct situation.

It is an empirical question whether the initial trigger for empathy being curiosity or resonance makes a difference in the accuracy of the empathy. Whether or not resonance occurs, however, some sense of having an emotional experience is part of empathy. Having an emotional experience while imagining another's fear helps guide me to imagine the threatening characteristics of things that I might otherwise not notice.[57]

In empathy, the physician's imagination and feelings work together to create a unified affective world that has the character of an experiential "totality."[58] This is like the totality created by a dancer, which cannot be reduced to a sum of discrete movements, as it adheres in her style, her timing, and her pauses between movements. Similarly, physicians express empathy not only by making accurate comments about a patient's feelings, but by their timing, vocal tones, pauses, and overall attunement to the affective style of a patient.

In closing, this emphasis on attunement fits with the empirical data emerging on empathy. For example, a recent study reported in the *Journal of the American Medical Association* closely observed patient–physician interactions and noted that before patients talk about emotional aspects of their history, they give hints and make gestures.[59] When physicians meet these hints with detached responses, no disclosure takes place. In contrast, when doctors attune to such clues nonverbally, patients communicate regarding emotionally laden topics and give fuller histories.[60] Insofar as empathy is a way of discerning when and what is salient in another's emotional communication, it performs a pre-logical, or extra-logical, "perceptual" activity. Insofar as patients come to physicians with more complexity than can fit on a preformatted check list, with problems that are still unrecognized or difficult to talk about, then empathy is critical for diagnosis and, therefore, for effective medical treatment.

This book began by noting that for physicians since the early twentieth century, medical effectiveness has depended upon pursuing correct diagnoses, and this aim has been equated with an interest in objective truth, as in science. This chapter focused on one critical use of empathy in medicine, which is to learn more about the patient's situation, as opposed to other, direct therapeutic uses of empathy. My argument against detachment as the most effective way to make diagnoses comes down to the claim that the pursuit of a correct diagnosis requires a *full*, as well as accurate, understanding of a patient's problems. Empathy involves discerning aspects of a patient's emotional experiences that might otherwise go unrecognized. Empathic communication enables patients to talk about stigmatized issues that relate to their health that might otherwise never be disclosed, thus leading to a fuller understanding of patients' illness experiences, health habits, psychological needs, and social situations. As for accuracy, to the extent that emotions focus attention, training physicians to be aware of the ways their emotions determine salience can also help them notice potential blind spots and biases. Empathy supplements objective knowledge, and the use of technology, and other tools for making accurate diagnoses.

A second use of empathy, explored in the next chapter, is to support patients in regaining psychological autonomy. Empathy helps patients process emotionally difficult information, such as hearing a diagnosis of cancer. This serves the important ethical goal of enabling patients to participate more fully in their treatment and in decisions about their futures.

Finally, by cultivating emotional reasoning, physicians can work to transform intense moments of emotional irrationality in medical practice, like that that occurred between Ms. G. and her physicians, into directly therapeutic interactions. The connection between projective identification—in which physicians inadvertently resonate with patients' fears and other painful emotions—and empathy will be explored in chapter 6. By contributing to diagnosis, patient autonomy, and therapeutic influence, empathy leads to more effective, and not just more pleasing, medical care.

NOTES

1. For evidence showing that bilateral emotional communication is therapeutic for patients, see, for example, Bertakis, Roter, and Putnam 1991; Levinson and Roter 1995; Blanck, Rosenthal, and Vannicelli 1986; and Harriagn et al. 1989. Medical researchers interested in psycho-neuroimmunology and alternative medicine are presenting an increasing body of empirical evidence showing the importance of emotional communication in healing. Recent studies have documented connections between patient–clinician relationships, emotions, treatment efficacy, and health outcomes. Rietveld and Prins documented an interaction between negative emotions and acute subjective and objective symptoms of childhood asthma. See Rietveld and Prins 1998. Kemeny and Dean reported that the bereavement process influences biological systems relevant to HIV pro-

gression, particularly a more rapid loss of CD4 T-cells. See Kemeny and Dean 1995. A later study showed men who engage in cognitive processing were more likely to find meaning from grieving and showed less rapid declines in CD4 T cell levels and lower rates of AIDS-related mortality, independent of health status at baseline, health behaviors, and other potential confounders. These results suggest that positive responses to stressful events, specifically the discovery of meaning, may be linked to positive immunologic and health outcomes. See Bower, Kemeny, and Taylor 1998. A structured psychiatric intervention for cancer patients was shown to significantly improve coping and affective disturbances. See Fawzy 1995, Fawzy and Fawzy 1998, and Fawzy et al. 1993. Similarly, support for bereaved parents improves psychosocial outcomes. See Heiney, Ruffin, and Goon-Johnson 1995. Frasure-Smith and her colleagues found that major depression, depressive symptoms, anxiety, and history of major depression all significantly and independently predicted cardiac events over the subsequent twelve months in patients admitted after an initial myocardial infarction. See Frasure-Smith, Lesperance, and Talajic 1995. Similar work has been done in heart failure and HIV/AIDS prevention, such as Krumholz et al. 1998 and Schwarzer, Dunkel-Schetter, and Kemeny 1994.

2. See, for example, a recent proposal for guidelines for medical school education: Medical School Objectives Writing Group 1999.

3. Basch 1983. After completing this book, a collected volume on empathy, gender and medicine that explores similar tensions over integrating affect into medical practice was brought to my attention. See More and Milligan, 1994.

4. According to Rosenberg and Towers, Blumgart's ideal physician does not relate to the patient "as one person to another, but rather collects 'data' from the patient's behavioral expressions for analysis and responses within the physician's own perspective. The physician is satisfied merely to observe the signs of the patient's illness, rather than to comprehend its experiential content." See Rosenberg and Towers 1986.

5. Osler 1963, p. 29.

6. For this definition of projection, see Guralnik 1972.

7. Even the term *point of view* is problematic, because how a patient feels in a situation includes vague, atmospheric feelings and moods as well as focused and pointed emotional judgments. This is discussed in chapter 3.

8. I reject the behaviorist claim that empathy is reducible to saying and doing things that make a person think he is being understood. My goal is to explain how genuine understanding is possible in the first place. For other issues regarding patient–physician trust, see Thom and Cambell 1997 and Hillman 1998.

9. Sheldon Margen, physician, professor, and former colleague of Aring's, personal communication, November 1999.

10. See Tugendhat 1986.

11. Wittgenstein's criticism of the Cartesian view of understanding as making "inner" comparisons is relevant to the prediction model of empathy. What kind of mental diagram or image could be the basis for comparing generalized knowledge of emotional states to an understanding of what an individual patient is feeling? The idea of an inner act does not *explain* how the empathizer is able to recognize and appreciate the experiential aspect of others' emotions. See Wittgenstein 1958. For a discussion of the distinction between the perspective of an agent, and that of an observer predicting another's actions see O'Shaughnessey, 1980.

12. Sawyier 1975.

13. I hypothesize that the fact that empathy involves multiple modes of cognition, including affective imagery and reflective thought, contributes to the "reality" of the object of empathy. This is based on the common observation that using multiple senses contributes to the reality of an object of perception.

14. Herman 1993b.

15. Although Lipps's definition of *Einfühlung* is the one cited by the *Oxford English Dictionary* today for empathy, he was not the first to use either the term or the concept of empathy. Aristotle spoke of "empathy" in the *Rhetorics*, referring to literary expressions such as Homer's description of an arrow flying "eagerly." Aristotle described this as "the practice of giving metaphorical life to lifeless things." See Aristotle, 1941: 11(1411 b 33 ff). This linguistic practice is not what we mean by "empathy." According to art historian Moshe Barasch, it was only during the late nineteenth century that the modern concept of empathy became the focus of aesthetic and psychological theory. First Robert Vischer coined the term *Einfühlung* in 1873, then Lipps developed the concept, as did Johannes Volkelt in Germany, Victor Basch in France, and Vernon Lee in England. See Barasch 1998. Lipps and William Wundt used the term *Einfühlung* in their "scientific" psychological work to describe the mental capacity to understand the psychic life of other persons. Lipps's statement that one could "fully comprehend" another's experience has behind it both the idea that empathy allows for a quasi first-person understanding of another and the idea that this understanding can, in principle, approach certainty. Schutz (and Dilthey before him) extended the idea that one could strive for certainty in one's knowledge of other persons to the idea that empathy could be the basis of a distinct form of reliable knowledge appropriate for the human sciences. See Lipps 1935. Also, see reference to Lipps in Hunsdahl 1967. For a discussion of Lipps's view of empathy as involving a complete merging with another, see Stein 1964 and Schutz 1967. For Dilthey on empathy, see Berger 1984.

16. As quoted in Barasch 1998, p. 111.

17. *Ibid.*, p. 184.

18. See Heidegger 1962. Heidegger offers a model for the kind of experiential "projection" of meaning that is essential for empathy. He argues that we do not first perceive things as meaningless sense data and then infer that they are objects that interest us, like tools, forests, and persons. Rather, the fact that as perceivers we attend to certain phenomena rather than others in meaningful, practically useful patterns reveals our capacity to "understand" the world pre-reflectively (section G, 150). The term *totality* does not refer to a collection of unrelated things. Heidegger refers to a web of mutually implicated things, like the totality of a painting. He claims that the particular tasks and objects of daily life are always understood in terms of a totality of involvements. His point is that understanding always takes place in a *context* of interests and projects (section G, 102–105). A second major point from Heidegger is that the cares and interests that provide a context for understanding something must be partially pre-reflective, or unthematized. The experience of being interested in something, which he calls a "fore-having," is necessary for recognizing a gap in one's grasp of the thing and hence for questioning and finally conceptualizing it. The idea that our pre-reflective attitudes toward things and other persons underlies the possibility of understanding them is the basis for Heidegger's claim that "moods" disclose reality. (section G, 150–152).

19. Interestingly, Heidegger takes the objective observer to be in a mood, one that *excludes* receiving affective input. He would see detached physicians as in a mood of excluding input.

20. Husserl 1977. See also Theunissen 1986.

21. I do not mean to suggest that cultural, linguistic, class, race, sex, and other differences are not crucial factors influencing doctor–patient communication. I discuss this in chapter 6. See Bach et al. 1999.

22. Deutsch 1970.

23. Fliess 1942.

24. Fenichel 1953.

25. Kohut 1959.

26. Because *Einfühlung* literally means "feeling into," and because we cannot literally feel into another's world, the concept functions as a metaphor. This topic requires further exploration, however, because empathy lies somewhere between directly observable mental processes, such as sense perception, and processes, such as repression, that are never themselves directly observed.

27. See for example, "The Unconscious,"(v. 14) and "Observations on Transference-Love" (v. 12) in Freud. Also see Freud 1959.

28. Rhetoricians depend upon this phenomenon when they deliberately use exaggerated expressions of anger and enthusiasm to incite a crowd. The reason for calling such responses "automatic" or "direct" is that they do not seem to rely on recollection, imagination, or any other mental act, other than noticing how another person feels.

29. Buie, for example, follows Freud (1892) in using the term "resonance feelings" to refer to those experiences in which one person's mood seems to be directly transmitted to another. See Buie 1981, pp. 297, 301.

30. Berger 1987, pp. 30–31.

31. Basch 1983, p. 105.

32. Kohut 1959.

33. Stein 1967, p. 13.

34. See Husserl on the "primordial" situation, in Husserl 1977.

35. Stein 1967, p. 13.

36. *Ibid.*, p. 16.

37. Stein addresses this point by agreeing with Lipps that it is *possible* to have an experience of oneness with another person. But she argues that such an experience cannot be the basis of empathy, since it actually presupposes empathy. For example, two soldiers on the front lines hear that the war is won. Both feel joy and relief and recognize each other's joy and relief. It is because they first *recognize* each other's feelings, as they actually share a situation, that they can have a "we" experience. See Stein 1967, p. 16.

38. Husserl 1977. Sartre was influenced by Husserl's idea that one can intuitively experience the absence of the other. However, Sartre took the more extreme position that awareness of another creates not only a sense of absence but a dynamic negation within one's own sense of being. See Sartre 1956.

39. Perhaps the phrase "putting oneself in another's shoes" is commonly understood as imagining what it is like to be in the patient's position, as opposed to imagining what it is like to be yourself facing her problems.

40. Guralnik 1972.

41. Katz 1983, p. 132.

42. Benner, Kidis, and Stannard 1999.

43. Note that Casey's definition of "imagining how" uses the term *projection* in a way that is distinct from Lipps's use. Unlike Lipps, Casey does not presuppose that in "imag-

ining how" one attributes one's personality to another. Rather, he has in mind a much more general meaning of projection, in which one fore-interprets, or provides a landscape upon which an experience can be made sense of.

44. Casey 1976, pp. 44–45.

45. *Ibid.*, p. 45.

46. Wollheim 1977.

47. This case is also presented (in a modified form) in Halpern, "*Using Resonance Emotions in the Service of Curiosity*," in Spiro, 1995.

48. Levenson and Ruef 1992.

49. A critique of the notion of empathy as an "as-if" experience is that this likens empathy to a kind of sentimentalism in which one is interested in one's own appreciation of another's emotions, rather than her suffering. Patricia Benner, personal communication, January 2000.

50. Langer 1953, p. 187.

51. *Ibid.*

52. According to the merging model, the physician views her imaginative portrayal of the patient as projecting *herself* into the patient's situation. Wollheim, speaking of the imagination in general, calls a *master thought* "the way in which we conceive or in which we represent to ourselves our mental processes, or the conception under which a mental process occurs." My view is that representing empathic imagining as a merging experience is a mistaken master thought. Rather, in imagining how it would feel to be in the patient's situation, the physician mixes her own affective repertoire with the patient's in order to fill out her portrayal of the patient's experience. Recall Edith Stein's (and Husserl's) point that the guiding intention of empathy is to grasp the situation of *another* person. This goal, with its explicit awareness of another's separateness, is the genuine master thought of empathy. See Wollheim 1967, p. 192, and Stein 1967.

53. To make this traditional conception of the interaction of thought and feeling more explicit, I elaborate on Wollheim's description of the features of imagining-how as the *inner* creation and performance of a play for an audience. The mistaken picture of empathic understanding is as follows: one's cognitive faculty writes and performs a play for an audience of two, including a translator who watches and translates the images into affective signals, and an affective audience, who respond mechanically to the signals. Given this picture, the possibility for appreciating new aspects of the drama cannot be explained. If the audience somehow gives emotional responses that translate into images that are appropriate for the next part of the drama, this would have to be a matter of sheer luck or be based on some magical, extrasensory capacity.

54. The possibility for new emotional meanings is illustrated by the fact that despite a certain patterning, people love and desire people and interests that are not exactly like their first love objects. Although psychoanalysis has emphasized the repetitive nature of human relationships, this should not be taken so literally as to imply exact repetition or complete stasis. See "Remembering, Repeating and Working-Through: Further Recommendations on the Technique of Psycho-Analysis II" in Freud 1966, pp. 147–156.

55. See Freud *The Interpretation of Dreams*, 534. In addition to the structural similarity between primary process thinking and imagining how another feels, other concrete similarities exist. For example, Freud points out that in dreams there is an elision of the "perhaps" that characterizes waking thoughts: If one is worried that someone is, perhaps,

angry at one, one does not dream that she might be angry, but that she *is* angry. The elision of the "perhaps" in dreaming corresponds to the elision of the hypothetical in empathy; empathy involves experiencing the announcement of another's feelings, rather than positing that, hypothetically, the other might feel a certain way.

56. Wollheim goes on to give the following example: A woman might experience a transient attraction to a woman whom she imagines her husband to be in love with, even though, lacking the appropriate sexual orientation, these feelings are not ones she would otherwise have. See Wollheim 1999, p. 10.

57. The claim that empathy involves having an emotional experience does require further empirical investigation because of some controversial findings. Research by Robert Levenson and Anna Ruef showed that both men and women attune emotionally (including the accompanying physiologic arousal) while empathizing with others. However, in long term relationships, women continue to have the same emotional attunement/arousal while empathizing with their husbands, but men do not necessarily experience emotional arousal while empathizing with their wives, even though they can still read their emotional states accurately. This important finding, in my view, does not disqualify my emphasis on emotional attunement in clinical encounters. First, in a long-term marriage, a husband may come to know so much about his wife's emotional patterns that he develops ways to predict her feelings, which is not the same process as experiencing empathy. Alternatively, there may be ways in which emotional arousal is systematically inhibited in such men toward their wives, so that they do empathize differently than normally occurs. However, despite all these possibilities, this research calls for more empirical examination of the role of emotional attunement in empathy. See Levenson 1992.

58. The sense of a "totality" or a "world" harkens back to Heidegger.

59. Suchman et al. 1997.

60. *Ibid.*

FIVE

Respecting Patient Autonomy: From Non-Interference to Empathy

This chapter applies the paradigm shift from detached concern to empathic engagement to the current ethical ideal in American medicine, that of respecting patient autonomy. This norm was expressed by the medical ethicist on Ms. G's medical team, who said, "Our ethical obligation here is to respect this patient's autonomy, which means her right to make up her own mind regarding her future without interference from us."

The norm of autonomy greatly influences current medical practice, although it is a recent ideal, emerging from the American medical ethics movement of the past thirty years.[1] The term autonomy refers both to a psychological capacity to make decisions that reflect one's own goals and an ethical ideal of individual self-determination. The term is used in medicine to describe an evolving set of patients' rights, extending from rights to determine what happens to one's own body, to rights to informed consent and refusal of treatment, to rights to participate more fully in medical decision making.[2] Many of these rights have emerged through lawsuits, and hence it is through a legalistic prism that physicians understand their obligations to respect autonomy.[3] Seeing autonomy as freedom from interference, they tend to overlook any positive role they might play in assisting patients to regain psychological autonomy. Respecting autonomy too often translates in practice into leaving patients alone, often without social supports to face difficult medical decisions.[4] In response to this, some feminists have criticized this ideal as neglectful and lacking an appreciation of the social basis of personhood and health values.[5]

My own view is that respecting patient autonomy is an important protection for patients lacking the voice and power to influence their own medical care.[6] However, promoting patient autonomy need not involve a policy of noninterference. One example of this is in disclosing cancer diagnoses. As recently as 1961, a study in the *Journal of the American Medical Association* reported that ninety percent of U.S. oncologists would not tell patients that they had cancer.[7] This paternalism has shifted as the ethical ideal of respecting patient autonomy has taken hold, and now it is the standard of care to inform patients. However, recent studies have shown that although patients are informed, they are also left feeling helpless and overwhelmed after hearing a difficult diagnosis. Research shows that empathic engagement helps patients hear and process such upsetting information.[8] Empathic engagement, rather than non-interference, I argue in this chapter, promotes patient autonomy. In particular, the mental conditions patients need to exercise autonomy are not determined only by events inside the patient's head but are influenced by emotional interactions with others, including physicians.

Respecting Autonomy: Beyond Non-Interference

Whether they realized it or not, Ms. G.'s physicians were guided by a norm of *negative* autonomy, or constraint from interfering with a patient's self-determination. This norm has been a central focus of the American bioethics movement over the last thirty years. This emphasis is a response to a long tradition of physician paternalism. The recent emphasis on negative autonomy grounds itself in a legalistic conception of the person as an independent agent who should not have treatment imposed on her by others.

At one level, the question of whether non-interference is appropriate when a patient is in obvious mental distress has already been faced in health law and in U.S. medical ethics. Note the famous case of Elizabeth Bouvia, a woman who had no terminal illness but who judged her life to be not worth living and asked to be allowed to refuse life-sustaining nutrition and die in the hospital with only comfort care.[9] Since Bouvia won her court case (though subsequently she decided not to end her life) frequent clinical cases have arisen of patients depressed about their quality of life (often including a social dimension) requesting that treatment be terminated. The literature about those cases has focused on assessing the capacity of such patients to make an informed treatment refusal.[10]

The criteria for capacity include not only whether a patient can literally state the risks and benefits of treatment, but also whether she can weigh and balance these risks as they apply to her own life.[11] Often, a treatment team will consult a psychiatrist to determine whether the patient's mental distress has rendered her unable to weigh and balance these risks appropriately. In Ms. G.'s case, for example, she was in an acute crisis and might very well have benefited from intensive psychotherapy, or even medication. She had previously benefited from psychiatric treatment when in a similar state of mind. This time, however, she refused to participate in such treatment.

If Ms. G.'s physicians had not been concerned with respecting her autonomy, they might have used a psychiatric diagnosis to seek a court hearing regarding her competency to refuse treatment.[12] A judge might have ordered that dialysis be continued temporarily against Ms. G.'s will, and that she be involuntarily admitted to a psychiatric hospital, even though no active treatment could have taken place there without her participation.

However, from an ethical standpoint, such an approach is problematic because the ethical basis for seeking a ruling on competency is a physician's judgment that a patient probably lacks decision-making capacity (competency is in legal language what capacity is in medical language). However, there are problems with each of the following statements: (1) Ms. G. lacked decision-making capacity and thus another person (a proxy) should have attempted to apply her previous, longstanding values and make the decision for her. (2) Ms. G.'s decision-making process demanded respect, and therefore her wish to terminate treatment (and therefore her life) should not have been interfered with.

Ms. G. was cognitively intact and could rationally state why she did not want further treatment. Therefore, even though she had psychiatric symptoms, it seemed that she did not lack decision-making capacity regarding specific treatment.[13] No evidence existed that she had psychotic symptoms, such as delusions of guilt, which sometimes accompany severe depression. Rather, like many suffering people in the hospital, she met the criteria for a psychiatric diagnosis yet was able logically to state her preferences regarding treatment. On the other hand, the problem with not challenging her capacity is that her practical reasoning was greatly impaired by her suffering. Although she was not crazy, her catastrophic thinking involved emotional irrationality.

Catastrophic thinking is commonplace in a setting of loss and trauma, and it is inappropriate to label every patient who feels hopeless about his future "incompetent." The term "patient" means "one who suffers," and what distinguishes suffering from states of discomfort is that one's personhood is somehow impinged upon. Ms. G.'s situation was complicated by her husband leaving, although her experience of a deep disruption in her preexisting life goals, and even her inability to form new ones, is not uncommon among patients. Losing mobility, vision, and sexual functioning and fearing further decline and death are all experiences that affect one's sense of agency, independence, and relationality. Recovering autonomy in the face of such losses, depending upon a person's internal strengths and external supports, may require as little as finding new goals or as much as finding a new sense of oneself as a center of initiative and efficacy. If respect for autonomy is to be genuinely relevant to patients, then it must be responsive to these experiential needs.

Suffering may impair people's self-efficacy as well as their ability to imagine goals for the future. Yet these two things are essential for exercising autonomy. Further, it is precisely when people are ill that they need these abilities, because medical decisions often rest on rethinking life goals. However, the rethinking needed involves grieving and other kinds of emotional as well as logical reasoning. That is, working through feelings of loss can help one arrive at a more realistic and authentic basis for making decisions than is possible by simply trying to detach from upsetting feelings.

Patients value being assisted in processing bad news emotionally so that they can genuinely regenerate goals. Yet, under the bureaucratic, marketplace, and legal influences in medicine, respecting autonomy increasingly consists of satisfying preexisting consumer preferences.[14] This precludes physicians helping patients go through a process of facing their illness and establishing treatment choices that reflect their personal values. It is not merely that a patient states a preference for one form of treatment over another, but also that the preference reflects the person's ends, or goals in shaping her own future, that make respect for autonomy crucial.

Despite the language of consumer preferences, physicians are in some way aware of the deeper motivation for respecting patient autonomy. If this were not the case, patients who stated that they had no preferences regarding serious medical decisions would not raise ethical concerns for doctors, but they do. In the treatment of breast or prostate cancer, physicians seek and take seriously even mild patient preferences for undergoing radical mastectomy versus lumpectomy and radiation versus cryosurgery. They do so because these alternatives seriously affect people's capacities for functioning in the world in distinct ways, and deciding which procedures are best requires personal value judgments about the relative importance of body image, sexual dysfunction, the risk of recurrence, and undergoing painful treatment. In such cases, doctors feel that patients should have an opportunity to form treatment goals that reflect their own values.

Although Ms. G.'s case was dramatic, most serious medical decisions involve value judgments that will shape patients' futures in various ways. Patients making daily medical decisions about treatments for heart disease, cancer, hypertension, and diabetes face significant trade-offs among risk of future mortality, living with dysfunction, living with pain, and tolerating side effects. Decisions of this sort involve choosing among different possible futures. Physicians concerned with patients' overall well-being cannot decide which type of loss and which type of benefit are of most value for individual lives. That is, these values are not reducible to a single, standardized scale of well-being. The deliberation involved in treatment trade-offs does not involve merely ascertaining an objective state of affairs but is a process of defining the best choice for the individual patient. The ideal of autonomy speaks to the value of the decision-making process itself.

The distinct value patient autonomy has, over and above individual well-being, is based on the importance we place on patients acting from their own conceptions of a worthwhile life in making practical choices that will seriously affect the kind of life they lead. However, as the case of Ms. G. illustrates, suffering impinges on one's capacity to think about one's future. The capacity to imagine oneself into new futures in the face of loss is central to decision-making in medicine, and the fact that no one else can determine what a person will consider worthwhile justifies making autonomy a cornerstone of medical ethics. Yet the mental freedom needed to deliberate wisely about her future is precisely what was lacking in Ms. G.'s case, and non-interference did nothing to restore it.

Patients facing serious medical decisions are likely to be in flux regarding their values because their life circumstances are changing so significantly. While the current emphasis on rights to non-interference protects patients who have preexisting preferences that remain unchanged, it does little for those whose psychological outlook is shifted by illness. Non-interference places the emotional processes involved in working through bad news and re-forming goals inside the patient's head, rather than in the social world, which includes the patient–physician relationship. To genuinely support autonomy in medicine requires a paradigm shift because patients, as sufferers, need assistance in regenerating the capacity to set future goals. Yet neither traditional medical paternalism nor a policy of detached non-interference meets this need. By understanding the emotional context shaping patients' medical decisions, physicians can genuinely assist patients to recover their capacities for autonomy.

Beyond Negative Autonomy: Kant on Deliberative Freedom

My emphasis on deliberative freedom as the basis of autonomy involves taking two steps beyond the current emphasis on negative autonomy as non-interference. The first step is to turn to a Kantian view that emphasizes a positive definition of autonomy by which a person generates ends, or goals, as a result of deliberation. I turn to Kant because his definition of autonomy is better suited to medicine than is the current emphasis on non-interference. He emphasizes the process of deliberation by which a person generates valued motives and actions. That is, for Kant, autonomy refers to a person's capacity to act in a way that is guided by the free and flexible use of her own reasoning, not to a person's liberty to do whatever she wants. For example, if a person wants to lie to avoid embarrassment, but her reasoning shows her that this is ultimately an inconsistent moral act, her autonomy expresses itself in her not doing what she wants to do, but in doing what she believes she ought to do. Kant's emphasis makes it possible to describe people who make tragic choices resulting in actions or outcomes they wish they did not have to face as acting autonomously. This is deeply relevant to patients, who often must decide among options that hardly reflect their wishes, and yet for whom it matters that they have the opportunity to deliberate regarding their own goals.

Kant defines autonomy as acting in accordance with one's reason, rather than as freedom from external constraints. In fact, Kant never talks about the freedom to do what one prefers without interference from others. He does not think autonomy is about expressing personal preferences in any way. Rather, Kant argues that exercising autonomy springs from a special kind of reasoning about what to do that is distinct from pragmatic reasoning about how to meet pre-existing preferences and needs. Reasoning about how to get what one already desires—means–ends reasoning—is something, he points out, that even animals seem able to do. Rather, Kant says that what is distinct about rational agents is their capacity to deliberate about ends—about what is worth doing and what is valuable. His idea is that persons use reasoning to stand apart from all their existing desires, emotions, and habits to generate effectively the motives (and actions) they believe they ought to have.[15]

Kant's focus on motives, or reasons for action, and his search for an incontestably good motive lead to his argument for the centrality of autonomy to morality. In the *Groundwork of the Metaphysics of Morals*, he writes:

> And I maintain that to every rational being possessed of a will we must also lend the Idea of freedom as the only one under which he can act. For in such a being we conceive a reason which is practical—that is, which exercises causality in regard to its objects. But we cannot possibly conceive of a reason as being consciously directed from outside in regard to its judgments; for in that case the subject would attribute the determination of his power of judgment, not to his reason, but to an impulsion. Reason must look upon itself as the author of its own principles independently of alien influences.[16]

Kant's conceives reason to be a cause that can liberate us from any of our preexisting dispositions, including suffering, so we can become authors of our own actions and determine our own goals for the future.

Despite Kant's divorce of rationality from emotion, his idea of conceiving of ourselves as free seems to me an important heuristic for what people who are suffering need to regenerate autonomy. In particular, I see at least two conditions for exercising autonomy that are relevant to patients facing decisions about their futures, both of which are inspired by Kant. The first is that a person needs to assume that her future is not wholly determined, so that her practical reasoning about what to do really matters. Second, she must see the world as sufficiently (if not perfectly) responsive to her own agency, so that generating a motive to act is seen both as necessary and not futile. These two conditions are essential for her to see her own reasoning regarding her choices as setting her on one causal path rather than another. That is, a person must assume that her actions are not wholly determined by causes beyond her own control and that a reliable connection exists between her deciding to act and causally affecting events in the social world. Suffering and the infantilizing experience of being in the hospital, however, disrupt both one's sense of having an undetermined future and one's sense of having causal efficacy.

For Kant, only the use of detached reasoning provides a sufficient basis for exercising autonomy. The power to spontaneously generate ends (or to determine goals), according to Kant, exists in the capacity to detach from all emotional and social influences. The kind of deliberation, Kant argues, that bestows moral worth on our actions is characterized by a person conceiving of herself as free to determine her own ends, based on Reason alone. By reason, Kant means Universal Reason, an unsituated and pure capacity to generate ideas.

Kant believed that we are never given an experience that shows that we are free to decide how to act, since our only knowledge of our experiences in the world is of ourselves as part of the nexus of psychological and physical causation. Yet, by using detached reason, persons can set aside these causal influences and envision goals that have independent moral worth.[17]

Kant's belief that one can generate ends spontaneously from a Universal Reason and his view of this as the positive essence of morality need to be justified. He thought it was possible for people to generate ends, or goals, independently of intuitions and empirical experience. He had already shown that fundamental aspects of perceiving reality, such as perceiving objects in space and time, were spontaneous productions of reason, rather than ideas that experience in the world causes us to have. That is, he believed that seeing events as linked spatially and temporally requires a mental construct of pure time and pure space that can never be observed empirically.[18] The Idea of freedom is to autonomy what underlying space and time concepts are to perception.

However, I disagree with Kant's equation of these detached conditions of autonomy with how people can motivate themselves to act. Rather, the deliberation that leads to action involves, among other things, socially situated emotional reasoning.

There is an important tension, then, in using Kantian thought in medical ethics. Kant's concept of autonomy as generative, the idea that through reasoning people can generate goals, is needed to supplant the non-interference model in medicine. On the other hand, for such ends to be the patient's own requires that the reasoning involved be socially and emotionally situated, an idea that Kant himself rejects, as I show in the following section. In order to resolve this tension, I turn later in the chapter to revisionist Kantians (who read Kant through a lens emphasizing social recognition and interdependence) to consider whether a view of autonomy based on emotional reasoning could be Kantian in spirit.

Autonomy versus Detachment

Kant's emphasis on detached reason as the basis of autonomy follows not simply from his notion of autonomy as conceiving of oneself as free, but also from his conception of reason as the same faculty in the theoretical and in the practical sphere. My goal is to sever the link between these ideas and rely only on the former. I reject his argument for the complete independence of practical reason from emotional needs.[19]

The idea of acting under a conception of oneself as free is based on a philosophically abstract model, and my goal is to integrate this account with the account of emotional communication and empathy developed in the previous chapters. In describing how suffering and grieving impinge on mental freedom, I argued that people develop emotional convictions about their futures (for example, Ms. G.'s conviction that she would always be alone and abandoned) that paralyze their capacity to imagine alternatives. A model of autonomy relevant to suffering must begin with how suffering impairs mental freedom and delineate what, in fact, regaining deliberative freedom requires.

Kant is in no way ignorant of human suffering and its impact on generating ends; he chooses, as one of his few illustrations of exercising autonomy, the case of a despondent and suicidal person. Yet Kant's purpose is to argue that a person's capacity to generate life goals, or "end-set," is practically (not just conceptually) independent from all affectivity. In the *Groundwork of the Metaphysics of Morals*, Kant talks about a man who feels utter despair and wants to end his life.[20] Importantly, Kant says nothing about the man's actual life—what happened to lead him to this state—or even the content of the man's specific painful thoughts. We do not know whether he feels rejected, like Ms. G., or guilty and furious with himself, or disillusioned in terms of his dreams and aspirations, or too anxious to enjoy anything—or any other complex of emotions that accompany suicidal states of mind. Kant takes none of these specifics to be pertinent to the moral issue. His point is that this man, who has no interest in living, still has the capacity to engage in autonomous deliberation. This deliberation requires detached reason alone. Specifically, it involves examining the principle characterizing his action to see if he could will it to be a universal law. To consider whether he endorses his goal of suicide from the perspective of universal reason, he formulates his end as a kind of law and considers its validity. He reflects on the maxim "It is permissible to take your own life when you no longer have an interest in living," and he finds that it cannot be universally valid.

It may seem that the ability of this man to engage in this kind of reasoning is unremarkable, since even in the most depressed emotional state one may still be cognitively intact. But Kant's claim goes much further: he claims that this reasoning is sufficient for the man to be *motivated* to refrain from suicide. That is, Kant's emphasis is on how reasoning can change a person's *will*, for Kant tells us that this exercise of detached reasoning is sufficient for the suicidal man to generate the new goal of continuing his own life.

My own reading of this case differs from Kant's in its aims as well as its conclusions. I take the man to be facing a genuine dilemma about whether his *own* future is worth living, whereas Kant is concerned with illustrating the power of moral motivation, the power of Universal Reason in the practical sphere. The detached reasoning Kant describes, in my view, is insufficient for the kind of psychologically rooted autonomy necessary for medical decision making. That is, even if the man were, on the basis of detached reasoning alone, capable of motivating himself against suicide (a claim that Bernard Williams and others have argued against), he still fails to express his autonomy in positive terms.[21] This failure is due to his lack of the two psychological conditions necessary for exercising mental freedom that I outlined above. He does not feel secure that his own immediate future is tolerable, and he has no valued goals that he can imagine implementing efficaciously. He therefore lacks a sense of his own future. His power to move himself by detached reason alone is insufficient for acting under a conception of himself as free.

This illustration is directly relevant to the dilemmas faced by patients today. For example, what process could give meaning or value to a cancer patient undergoing the hardship of noxious chemotherapy? The value of treatment depends on the person determining that it meets his own goals for the future. In facing cancer treatment decisions, the ability to take risks depends on forming goals that make it personally worthwhile to undergo hardship. If a person were emotionally out of touch with all that moves him, as Kant's suicidal man is, it is unclear what could form the rationale for going through cancer treatment. From a constricted emotional state in which one lacks all hope or personal interest in one's future, one may decide to fulfill the impartial duty to refrain from suicide. Whatever freedom this decision reflects, however, will not serve patients who need to make choices among distinct benefits and burdens, each of which requires feeling one's way imaginatively into an unknown future.

The conception of autonomy as involving deliberative freedom is relevant to medicine only insofar as it points to a patient's capacity to imagine her *own* goals for the future. The capacity to make use of detached reason to commit to impersonal goals is not the proper capacity for this kind of autonomy. On one hand, the demands of Universal Reason are too strong. As Kant argues, from the standpoint of Universal Reason suicide is impermissible. On the other hand, detached reason is too barren for envisioning a future with the real effects of illness and treatment, yet worth living. This kind of imaginative filling-in involves emotional reasoning.

Detached reason is insufficient for helping patients regain mental freedom. Yet Kant's belief that it is genuinely possible for persons to act under a conception of themselves as free serves as an important ground for respecting patient autonomy. In the next section I explore the role of empathy in this process.

Suffering, Empathy, and the Interpersonal Basis of Autonomy

Kant equates the freedom that makes decision-making autonomous with reason's "independent" nature. He describes reason as *selbständig*, a term used to describe a piece of furniture that stands by itself. However, as I argue in the next section, Kant's idea of reason as setting its own ends does not require that people act in social isolation.[22]

Suffering creates special conditions that make an interpersonal model for regenerating autonomy preferable. In suffering, expectations about the reliability of the world and of one's capacity to achieve any of one's goals can be destroyed. Ms. G., for example, lacked a basic feeling that her immediate future was tolerable. Her certainty that her future was hopeless impaired her capacity for autonomy. She was unable to see her future as livable because of a deep conviction that she would be perpetually abandoned.

I have already described the cognitive features of concretized states of mind like Ms. G.'s and shown how such emotional convictions preclude imagining alternatives. As I argued, the openness or potential that one attributes to one's future is ordinarily colored by affects. This is apparent during intense emotional states, such as falling in love, in which the world and one's own future become suddenly rich with possibilities. What distinguishes concretized states lacking mental freedom, like Ms. G.'s, is that they are impervious both to the normal ebb and flow of emotions and to other ideas and new information.[23] For example, while romantic love may often be nearsighted, only concretized love resists negative information against the beloved (or the beloved's devotion) to the point of appearing to be "blind." Emotions in general influence whether we feel it is worth forming goals and whether we believe others will be receptive, indifferent, or rejecting.

The problem for people who are suffering is not just that they cannot imagine future goals that are several steps away, but that they also lack enough security and comfort to feel a sense of ongoingness into the immediate future. Without the sense that life is currently tolerable, practical reasoning loses its point. There is no reason to form any intention other than to bring about the termination of one's suffering—and one's existence. Assisting people like Ms. G. to recover their autonomy requires alleviating suffering sufficiently that it is tolerable to go on living another moment. This, in turn, demands empathy for the specific threats or harms that most impinge upon a patient's experience, whether it be physical pain, fear of an imminent painful procedure, or a terrible feeling of rejection. This kind of specificity guides both hospice workers and psychiatrists who help suicidal patients, both of whom describe the need to help patients feel safe and secure enough to find their immediate future tolerable.

It is a large step, however, from alleviating suffering so that a patient can imagine going on to the next moment of her life to helping someone envision a longer-term future. There are at least three ways that physicians may be able to assist patients in this difficult process. First, for a person in a state of intense suffering, wandering through her imaginative world feels as frightening as walking through the most threatening real-world situation. The function of empathy in such cases is not merely to diagnose a person's condition, but to give her the sense that she is not alone with her thoughts. The goal for the doctor, however, is not to merge, or over-identify, with the sufferer, not to act is if she and the patient are in the same situation, but to recognize the threats the patient feels. To use philosopher Susan Brison's analogy, the patient is akin to a person recovering from a street assault, and the doctor is the imaginative equivalent of the secure and trusted friend who walks with her through the streets of her town at night until she regains her sense of security.[24] As I have already argued, the doctor who is engaged empathically can do what a detached listener cannot—follow or accompany someone through the specific terrain of her interior world.

Feeling so accompanied is healing in part because it helps make it possible for the sufferer to feel the full scope of intensely aversive affects, such as overwhelming grief or fear. For many patients, simply being able to cry and otherwise express strong feelings while feeling accompanied is therapeutic. Freud conceived of this as a healing "abreaction," like lancing a boil of repressed emotion, a view that has been criticized as overly mechanistic.[25] However, his view is only a more modern version of a long tradition in medicine of psychological healing that emphasizes catharsis.[26] What has been emphasized less, but appears central to the restoration of autonomy, is the second step in healing. An empathic listener, by expressing her own curiosity, can generate a healing curiosity in another.

Engaging empathically with Ms. G. might have enabled her to rediscover her own curiosity about her concretized hopelessness. That is, whereas sympathetic identification involves joining someone in concretizing the hopelessness they feel, empathy makes it possible to move through a concretized state to something else. The function of empathy is not to project one's own fearful experiences onto another person. Rather one gains an experiential understanding of what moves another person by imaginatively following her affective ebbs and flows. Clinical empathy, as opposed to Lipps's view of empathy for a work of art,[27] is not about intensely holding on to one affective moment, but about apprehending the complex layering of another person's emotions. As I will describe in the next and last chapter, this process involves using curiosity not only to fill in imaginative details, but also to challenge apparent concretizations.

Most importantly, such curiosity needs to arise in a state of affective attunement with the person suffering and not in a state of detachment. Otherwise, the person is at risk of being treated as a curiosity. Curiosity in a context of affective engagement allows someone simultaneously to take herself seriously and yet to become curious about her convictions about the future. Ms. G.'s concretized belief that her future was hopeless denied the temporality and ambivalence characterizing realistic emotional assessments. Most likely, as she recovered from her traumatic news, she would have experienced emotional fluctuations and even contradictory feelings about her future.

For Ms. G. to have developed a healing curiosity about her own reactions this curiosity would have needed to be empathic and not self-critical. That is, it would have been necessary for her to respect the seriousness of the threats she faced and not devalue her own fear, even as she developed some sense of perspective beyond the state of terror she was in.

Respecting another as an end-setter begins with understanding her present state of mind, including the affective attitudes that shape her interests and beliefs. Without such understanding, we cannot see why another's ends have value, unless we project our own ends onto them. Understanding someone in this way is very different from exhorting someone to be in some more suitable state of mind.

A third facet of using empathy in support of autonomy has to do with the interpersonal support necessary for developing a sense of self-efficacy. People imagining new goals for themselves need to feel that they can be effective in the social world—that they can enlist others' participation in achieving their own ends. To consider this issue, I look to accounts of how children develop self-efficacy in the first place. However, this is not meant to suggest that adult patients are to be infantilized, that physicians are to be in any sense parental, or that adults have the plasticity and openness of children. Rather, the point of such accounts is to show that at least the initial development of self-efficacy is an interpersonal process in which other people's recognition of a person's agency, or the lack thereof, is highly influential.[28]

For children to develop a sense of initiative, parental recognition of small attempts at autonomy is crucial. Parental hopefulness or fearfulness regarding the child's future has lasting impact. But even this way of framing the situation is too cognitive, because it is not just that parents convey the *idea* of efficacy to their children. Rather, by being responsive to their children's initiatives through nonverbal and verbal communication as well as affective resonance, parents influence their children's states of being—the hopefulness, tentativeness, anxiety, or fearfulness that make it possible for children to initiate activity or learn passivity.

In families where children are neglected or abused, children often develop a sense that they cannot do anything to create a future in which their own goals and projects will somehow be realized in the world.[29] Although the impact of chronic trauma is profound, therapists have been able to work successfully with children who have endured trauma to help them regenerate a conception of having their own futures. The major therapeutic intervention is to accompany the child empathically as he recollects disowned affects of fear or terror. When the patient is still a child and cannot simply put his experience into words, the mode of communication is play therapy. Children who have been traumatized tend to repeat traumatic experiences in their imaginative play. The therapist can help the child recognize what is being expressed in the play. The child then may directly feel fear or grief in the presence of the therapist for the first time. Once these feelings are in the room, children are able to use play to work on their threatening beliefs—thus loosening the hold of the conviction that they are going to be killed, or are going to die, or will be abandoned in the future.

Adults repeat their traumas just as children do, and in the highly intense setting of the hospital it is not unusual for each member of a treatment team to reenact personal conflicts without being aware of it. That is, patients who feel deeply hopeless or fearful can evoke similar states in their caregivers. As long as doctors and nurses remain unaware of this process, their own responses may unwittingly reinforce their patients' feelings. Ms. G.'s suffering could not be kept somewhere in her "head," but rather was manifest in her entire interaction with her treatment team. Although she asked to be left alone, yelling "Get out of here!" her agony was over the fact that she felt utterly abandoned. Her silent screaming, her frightened withdrawal into a fetal position, and her mental image of her husband saying that he could never love her again because of her deformity also communicated the message, "I am alone! I have been left to die!" If her doctors had engaged empathically with Ms. G., they might have become conscious of how strongly they identified with her hopelessness and become curious about her outlook—instead of simply colluding in her decision to die.

This case illustrates a key point about autonomy: non-interference is, in fact, not benign, because the mental freedom to imagine one's own future often comes not from some process inside one's head, but from processes in the social world. It is through emotional communication starting in early infancy that we develop a sense of agency and efficacy, a lifelong process. When one's identity and goals are stable, a person can be resilient and emotionally independent and withstand social rejection or neglect without being seriously affected. However, when someone's entire sense of self is disrupted, as occurs with suffering and trauma, the impact of not being empathized with can be very severe. Susan Brison describes this process:

> Primo Levi recalls a dream in which he is telling his sister and others about Auschwitz and they are completely indifferent, acting as though he is not present. Many others had a similar dream. . . . Why is it so horrifying for survivors to be unheard? Not to be heard means that the self that the survivor has become does not exist. Since the earlier self died, the surviving self needs to be known and acknowledged in order to exist.[30]

The question of what counts as acknowledgment of the surviving self is an interesting one. This term might be taken to imply intellectual recognition, but what Holocaust survivors needed was more than simply having others believe that they went through horrors. Rather, these survivors overwhelmingly surrounded themselves with others who knew about what it was like to experience the Holocaust.[31] Brison similarly describes how rape survivors benefited from group therapy. Some of the members of the group who could not access overwhelming feelings, such as intense anger at the assailant, empathized with other people's predicaments, felt vicarious anger, and then came to recognize their own anger.[32]

What relevance does the role of empathizing with other survivors have for Ms. G.? She was in the kind of catastrophic emotional state in which being able to empathize with herself through vicarious identification would have been helpful. The distance created by empathizing with another person enables one to grasp that the unthinkable has happened without feeling overwhelmed by catastrophic emotions. Child psychiatrists often tell their young patients stories about another child's experience. This technique introduces emotionally intense material that the child can then empathize with and gradually apply to her own life.

How this applies in the medical setting is, of course, problematic. It would certainly have been odd for the members of Ms. G.'s medical team to sit down beside her and tell her about their own or other patients' personal losses. Yet it is no less problematic that her caregivers tried to manage their anxiety about her situation by detaching and spending as little time with her as possible. It seems obvious, once the norm of non-interference had been replaced by an ideal of empathy, that Ms. G.'s situation would have evoked fears of abandonment in all the people who cared for her. Further, if her doctors, having consciously recognized their own emotions, had made acknowledging comments regarding common experiences of loss, perhaps this would have helped Ms. G. feel less like a pariah. A fundamental, unacknowledged emotion at the core of Ms. G.'s suffering was a feeling of shame. Her physicians failed to recognize this and therefore, by their detachment, exposed her to ongoing shame, a most intolerable emotion.

This surely made it more difficult for her to recover autonomy. Shame prevents a sense of self-efficacy, leading to a powerful feeling of be ng "unselved." This emotional state, in particular, requires subtle empatnic attention, because sympathizing or otherwise intervening with patients at such moments can exacerbate shame. Recall how my pity for Mr. Smith made him feel ashamed. On the other hand, however difficult it is to bear, shame is a transient emotional state and does not signify a lasting incapacity to exercise autonomy. An individual can quickly shift from shame to regain a sense of self, given the right interpersonal circumstances. Groups for people suffering illness and trauma can be especially helpful in this regard. Empathizing with members of the group allows patients to see other people as vulnerable without blaming them or feeling ashamed of them. This may help each person tolerate her own vulnerability without overwhelming shame.

In the next chapter I will describe how physicians can shift from projective identification, as occurred when her doctors concretely believed that Ms. G.'s life was intolerable, to acknowledging such emotions and helping patients regain a sense of self. Perhaps if Ms. G.'s physicians had been consciously aware that they were deeply affected by her fear and shame, rather than seeing her situation as concretely hopeless, they might have sought to engage with her for a period of time without resorting to increasing her morphine dosage.

This leads me to return to the two problematic options that seemed to present themselves in Ms. G.'s case: to view *her* as lacking decision-making capacity or to view her decision-making *process* as commanding respect. The problem is that these possibilities are not exhaustive. Ms. G., as an individual, did not lack decision-making capacity: she could speak for herself, but needed support. As it happened, her decision-making process took place under the impulsion of her catastrophic feelings of shame and abandonment, which influenced her physicians as well. Given a better process of communication, she might well have been able to exercise autonomy.

How is this emphasis on the interpersonal conditions of decision-making compatible with a philosophical concept of autonomy? I turn now to revisionist readings of Kantian autonomy to show that by supplanting Kant's emphasis on detached reasoning with interpersonal models of agency, empathy can be seen to play an essential role in respecting autonomy.

Kantian Theory and Positive Obligations to Share Ends

First, is there some contradiction in claiming that exercising autonomy depends upon social conditions? No, not even from Kant's viewpoint. Kant does not argue that autonomy *requires* acting in the absence of all emotional support from others. The emphasis on non-interference in recent medicine is not Kantian. Rather, Kant sees a certain kind of mutuality as important for respecting persons. He emphasizes that in order to genuinely respect others' ends, we need to do more than let others be. We need to share in those ends in some positive sense:

> Now humanity could no doubt subsist if everybody contributed nothing to the happiness of others but at the same time refrained from deliberately impairing their happiness. This is, however, merely to agree negatively and not positively with humanity as an end in itself unless everyone endeavors also, so far as in him lies, to further the ends of others. For the end of a subject who is an end in himself must, if this conception is to have its full effect in me, be also, as far as possible, my ends.[33]

Two philosophers, Christine Korsgaard and Barbara Herman, provide alternative ways of reading Kant as envisioning positive engagement with others as a necessary aspect of respecting them as end-setters. Korsgaard de-emphasizes reason's *selbständig* nature and focuses on Kant's conception of an idealized community of rational agents, the "kingdom of ends." She argues that Kantian moral agency involves built-in role-reversal, or reciprocity. In order for the Kantian agent to consider himself a legislator in a kingdom of ends, he needs to consider himself as sharing in the ends of others:

> In order to make the ends and reasons of another your own, you must regard her as a source of value, someone whose choices confer worth upon their objects, and who has the right to decide on her own actions. In order to entrust your own ends and reasons to another's care, you must suppose that she regards you that way, and is prepared to act accordingly. People who enter into relations of reciprocity must be prepared to share their ends and reasons, to hold them jointly, and to act together. Reciprocity is the sharing of reasons, and you will enter into it only with someone you expect to deal with reasons in a rational way. In this sense, reciprocity requires that you hold the other responsible.[34]

Korsgaard's emphasis on reciprocity, rather than the *selbständig* nature of the moral agent, suggests a Kantian account of what was missing in the treatment of Ms. G. In agreeing to "respect" her wishes for noninterference, her physicians did not fully share in her ends as a moral agent. Because she was in a reactive rather than proactive state, her normal context for setting ends had been ripped apart. To genuinely determine her own ends would have required her to develop a new context for acting in the world. And she had not even begun to engage in this kind of regenerative work.

Absent Ms. G.'s own capacity to formulate ends in this active way, those attempting to treat her with respect could not actually do so. Respect for others requires regarding them as capable of deliberative freedom. That is, respect for others involves what Kantian morality already requires of oneself: that we regard the other not merely as a determined being affected by circumstances, but as a center of initiative and value. Ms. G.'s primary care internist, moved by sympathy, appreciated her suffering but did not respect her agency by holding her responsible for her own ends. The rest of the medical team attempted to respect her wishes without judging or understanding them, which fails to meet Korsgaard's basic requirement of reciprocity. No one shared in her ends in the fuller sense of understanding her passive experience of suffering while holding in mind her potential as an agent.

So the problem in Ms. G.'s case was that by permitting (and enabling) her treatment refusal and death, her doctors were still not respecting her autonomy. Neither choice that her physicians considered, given the lack of emotional communication that occurred, respected her autonomy.

What if better communication, including effective empathy, had occurred, and after a period of serious reflection she had decided that her life was no longer worth living? Could her physicians have respected this choice? This question illustrates the point of making respect for patient autonomy central to medicine. We expect physicians to respect patients' goals even when their values differ radically from the physicians' own.

One limitation of Korsgaard's view is that the emphasis on sharing ends seems to imply that people actually must hold the same goals to respect each other, which would mean physicians respect patients only insofar as they personally value the same goals as do their patients. For, according to Korsgaard, the rationality of another's ends is part of what I am to be moved by in respecting them, and, conversely, I have obligations to promote those ends of theirs that I can rationally affirm.

It is unclear how a Korsgaardian reading, which emphasizes the necessity of valuing another's ends in order to respect her agency, can do justice to situations in which physician and patient disagree on substantive ends. This calls into question exactly what Korsgaard means by saying that respect involves being moved by the rationality of another's ends. The term *rationality* here cannot just mean seeing that there is a reason that this person has these ends, but rather seems to require seeing the reason *in* the person's ends. But if this means being moved by the same ends, this is too strong a requirement to preserve room for the profound disagreements that physicians have with patients about when life is worth living.

Barbara Herman offers an alternative reading, in which the requirement is to support the process by which another deliberates, rather than share the other's ends. Herman thus delineates a commitment to aid others that arises because of an obligation to respect their autonomy, distinct from any obligation to value or promote others' particular ends or projects:

One might view the idea of taking another's ends as my own not in the sense that I should be prepared to act in his place (I act for him; I get for him what he wants when he cannot). Rather, in the sense that I support his status as a pursuer of ends, so that I am prepared to do what is necessary to help him maintain that status. We might say "I help him pursue-his-ends" and not "I help him in the pursuit of his ends." This interpretation acknowledges the other as a rational, autonomous agent in a way that the "community of ends" interpretation does not. It leads to the view that the well-being of another is something more than the (passive) satisfaction of his desires. What I support is the other's active and successful pursuit of his self-defined goals. I promote another's well-being or happiness by supporting the conditions for his pursuit of ends. That is, what I have a duty to do is to contribute to the meeting of his true needs when that is not within his power. On this interpretation, then, in taking another's ends as my own or his happiness as an obligatory end, I acknowledge him as a member of a community of mutual aid.[35]

After reading Korsgaard and Herman, the ethical problem with Ms. G.'s case emerges more clearly. That is, although Ms. G.'s preferences were followed and she was not interfered with, her reasoning was not genuinely respected. Even though the substance of her decision, her choice to die, could have been a proper object of respect, the process by which she arrived at it was problematic. There are other cases in which patients have refused life-sustaining treatment as the outcome of a process of deliberation reflecting their own values, a process that commands respect. But, in the case of Ms. G., her unrelieved psychological suffering impaired her ability to deliberate in a way that could confer value on her decision. By ignoring how her emotional state limited her capacity to envision her future and acceding to her preferences, her physicians did not genuinely respect her as a person.

If respect for autonomy involves a commitment to understanding patients' affective worlds, how far have we come from a practical emphasis on non-interference? Let us return to the moral dilemma in the case of Ms. G. How could her physicians have supported her empathically when she did not want to talk about her experiences? Did my question violate her autonomy, even if, in general, empathy is a necessary foundation for respecting others as end-setters? This case involves a fundamental ethical dilemma between a patient's right to privacy and a physician's obligation to understand a patient's reasons for refusing treatment. Just as a physician owes a patient respect for her dignity in examining her body, and should not expose her body to others, physicians owe patients respect for their mental privacy. For this reason, to ask patients questions repeatedly, or refuse to give them a break when they no longer want to talk, or worse yet, threaten them with coercive treatment unless they talk, would violate their dignity in the same way that unwarranted touching would.

In the language of rights and duties, to which medical ethics is often reduced, doctors have a duty to seek to understand the affective worlds of their patients, and therefore patients do not have a fundamental right to non-interference. But patients do not have a duty to explain themselves to their physicians. Rather, physicians have a duty to seek to understand the specific affective worlds of their patients, especially when they are suffering. This is not to say that some other duty may not conflict with, or even override, this duty. For example, although I do not believe medical practice can be guided by a duty of non-maleficence, because many therapeutic treatments cause transient harm, there is certainly a duty to avoid gratuitous harm.

My question, "What besides your body is hurting you?" led Ms. G. to talk about what she intensely both wanted and did not want to talk about. From one point of view, this question did gratuitous harm, because Ms. G. never benefited from talking to me (given her immediate death). A more empathic question for Ms. G. would have focused more closely on her actual state of mind, which involved a conflict between talking and not talking, thinking and not thinking. Asking about that ambivalence might have left her more options to pace the conversation with me.

From another perspective, the question as asked could have started a therapeutic process. Even in cases of terrible trauma, people have an ongoing interest in telling about or otherwise expressing their pain and need only to see that their physicians can genuinely withstand hearing about it. For example, Ms. G. did respond to my curiosity by beginning to tell me, with urgency, what had happened to her. But as she became aware of this she felt so much pain and fear that her intense feelings shifted towards anger at me. Yet her yelling at me was already the beginning of her regenerating a sense of her own agency—she was indignant, she had been wronged, and she had her own reasons to yell at me. The last chapter will explore how such moments of anger and upset, which doctors try to avoid, can be therapeutic opportunities. Had Ms. G. not died so quickly, her venting intense anger at me, if understood empathically, might have been the beginning of her recovery.

Kant's conception of end-setting lacks a developmental view of human agency. Recovering from suffering and imagining a worthwhile future is not a solitary task. Suffering needs to be alleviated before a person can regenerate a robust sense of her own efficacy. Alleviating suffering occurs through, among other things, emotional communication. People often express their pain in such a way as to have an emotional effect on other people. By refusing to let patients affect them, physicians cut off communication. On the other hand, as is commonly observed in psychotherapy, a clinician's empathy at such moments has a large effect in enabling patients to find some relief from the stranglehold of intense fear or despair.[36] In the final chapter I will describe developmental models that show the therapeutic power physicians gain by learning to endure, rather than flee from, the emotional impact patients like Ms. G. have on them. These models aim to redress a fundamental way that detachment abandons patients.

In summary, medical ethics needs a positive conception of respect for autonomy to correct for the legal model of non-interference. Kant's emphasis on deliberative freedom is a good candidate. Although Kant pictures the capacity to generate ends as springing from detached, *selbständig* reason, we can reject this picture by considering that under conditions of suffering, people depend upon empathic recognition to achieve freedom from catastrophic emotions. The use of empathy in the service of restoring autonomy is distinct from sympathetic identification, which supplants the patient's ends with ends defined by the physician. To genuinely respect Ms. G.'s autonomy would have required engaging empathically with full openness to the possibility that she still might refuse dialysis. If I had worked with her longer, such a choice would have been one I would have found personally upsetting but would have needed to respect.

The Complex Relationship Between Empathy and Respecting Autonomy

At the beginning of this book, it may have puzzled the reader that a text emphasizing empathy also focuses on autonomy, since there is a tension in medical ethics between patient autonomy and more relational models of care. However, this text has assumed certain connections between the two. In contrast to long-standing forms of emotional healing that bypass the patient's collaboration, such as the use of physician authority for persuasion or reassurance, the aim of empathy is to grasp the patient's own perspective. In clinical practice, an empathic physician and a physician guided by the ideal of respecting autonomy will ask the same kinds of questions of patients: What do you think is wrong? What do you think will happen? What do you fear most? What do you hope for?[37] What do you want out of treatment? What do you want to avoid? The emphasis on personal meaning links empathy with the goal of respecting patient autonomy.

My account of empathy as therapeutic has been influenced by a focus on helping patient's regain personal meaning.[38] This presumes that the locus of suffering is not the body as a biological entity, but the person as an existential being facing a loss of meaning and purpose.[39] However, empathy is needed for reasons other than for helping patients regain autonomy. From patients' perspectives, survival and the alleviation of pain and distress usually come before striving for self-determination. Further, sometimes patients do not want to shoulder too much responsibility for medical decisions.

Atul Gawande, a Harvard surgeon, eloquently describes how patients sometimes want their physician to make a critical medical decision for them, as he wanted the pediatrician to make decisions for him when his baby daughter was critically ill. This can be seen, technically, as exercising autonomy, because the patient *asks* the doctor to decide for him, but it is also an expression of an emotional need not to bear the responsibility for a threatening decision.[40] Exhorting patients to make their own decisions in such cases is akin to Christian Barnaard's error in exhorting Phillip Blaiberg to "take this plane up with me," a projection of the doctor's (or the ethicist's) agenda onto the patient.

Interpersonal aspects of healing unrelated to promoting autonomy, including the use of therapeutic touch and guided imagery, are beneficial in alleviating suffering. Sadly, in Ms. G.'s case, the only genuine relief I managed to offer her was the use of guided imagery to help her momentarily forget her suffering. Further, although empathy makes use of nonverbal communication and resonance, I have insufficiently examined the direct healing influence of the nonverbal aspects of empathy—including the benefits of simple attention. It is often a physician's message that she will not abandon a patient, rather than helping the patient articulate her feelings, that plays the most therapeutic role.[41] The final chapter, on fitting empathy into medical practice, explores how empathy can be therapeutic even when little verbal communication exists between a patient and a physician.

NOTES

1. Few other cultures prioritize truth-telling and respect for autonomy. See Glick 1997, Good 1991, Good et al. 1990, and Lind et al. 1989.

2. See Katz 1984.

3. *Ibid.* See also Ladd 1979.

4. Bioethicists have critically evaluated the minimalistic expectations of current patient–physician interactions. See Brody 1987 and Brody 1990.

5. There are diverse feminist critiques of autonomy. Some argue that the norm of autonomy is too barren and reductive of human relationships and needs to be left behind in favor of a more relational ethical ideal. Others argue that autonomy is a developmental ideal that presupposes supportive relationships. See, for example, Brison 1996 and Meyers 1997.

6. One formulation of respect for autonomy is that patients, as persons, should not be treated as a means to others' ends. This is a crucial formulation for a feminist bioethics, as physicians have traditionally judged women's health needs according to the functions women were thought to serve for others. This formulation of respecting autonomy as not treating people merely as means, but always regarding them as "ends-in-themselves," comes directly from Kantian moral theory. See Kant 1964.

7. Oncologists' attitudes about truth telling have shifted remarkably over time. See Oken 1961, Holland et al. 1987, and Novack et al. 1979.

8. For research on patient–physician communication and teaching physicians how to be empathic in communicating "bad news," see Ptacek and Eberhardt 1996 and Ptacek et al. 1999.

9. See Annas 1984, Annas 1984b, and Kane 1985.

10. Appelbaum, Lidz, and Meisel 1987.

11. *Ibid.*

12. In this case, she met criteria for an "adjustment disorder," which applies to patients in distress for too short a time to be labeled as having "major depression." See *American Psychiatric Association: Diagnostic and Statistical Manual of Mental Disorders*, Fourth Edition. Washington, DC: American Psychiatric Association, 1994.

13. Determinations of capacity are, by medical practice standards and law, to be restricted to a patient's understanding of each specific treatment decision, and not to reflect some global judgment. See Ross and Halpern 1995.

14. Recently, philosophers, including Harry Frankfurt, have developed an influential account of freedom of the will that emphasizes not the openness of a person's options but rather her capacity to endorse reflectively her own goals (Frankfurt would say "desires"). See Frankfurt 1988; see also Farber, Novack, and O'Brien 1997.

15. Philosophers debate the plausibility of Kant's claim that detached deliberation is sufficient to motivate action. See Herman 1993a. Recently, philosophers have disagreed about whether Kant's stoic view of emotions is central to his philosophical claims or can be, as I have suggested, set aside, leaving some of his important contributions intact. For

an account of the centrality of Kant's stoic view of the emotions, see particularly Schott 1988. For a creative use of Kantian theory that integrates more recent work on emotions, see Velleman 1999.

16. Kant 1964, p. 448.

17. In fact, reasoning about personal goals, in the way that patients need to, is for Kant not even an example of reasoning about ends, but rather is an example of reasoning about means to the end of personal happiness, a contingent and morally insignificant goal.

18. Kant 1965.

19. Many philosophers have entirely rejected Kant's notion of pure practical reason because they find implausible the claim that the same spontaneity that enables reason to order knowledge in the theoretical sphere is a sufficient basis for causal efficacy in the practical sphere. Kant's view of detached reason is of a reason detached not only from particular passions but also from all empirical motives. However, as many philosophers have pointed out, this view seems to presuppose that there really is a self existing outside all experience, a noumenal self, that is the source of one's agency. This metaphysical assumption has been frequently attacked because it seems to contradict Kant's argument that the concept of causality is an intellectual schema brought to experience by the human knower. That is, how can one give content to the idea of a kind of agency beyond all the conditions by which we know causality in the empirical world? To remain agnostic regarding this issue, I read Kant's discussion of pure practical reason in a deflationary way, to mean only that reason detaches from emotions and interests, not necessarily that reason acts from outside empirical causation. It is this more restricted claim about emotional detachment that I take issue with. See Herman 1993.

20. Kant 1964.

21. Williams 1981.

22. To dichotomize interpersonal and solitary agency is imprecise. A person can be alone and yet empathize with herself, having been subject to empathy in the social world, so that a solitary agent can benefit from modes of deliberation that I label, for heuristic reasons, interpersonal.

23. Stolorow et al. 1987.

24. Brison 1996.

25. Jonathan Lear traces the concept of catharsis from Aristotle to Freud. See Lear 1988 and Lear 1995.

26. On the tradition of catharsis in medicine, see Jackson 1992.

27. Lipps 1935.

28. Empathy enables new experiences to emerge and be integrated into a person's sense of self via processes of recognition and acknowledgment of recognition. Various philosophical accounts exist of the role of recognition by another in constituting one's own sense of self and agency. A most influential thinker on the subject was Hegel. He describes a complex process in which, by recognizing an other view of it, consciousness can experience its own subjectivity from an objectifying distance, and thereby repossess it, acknowledging its existence in the world. See Hegel 1977. An important limitation in applying Hegel here is that his account abstracts from discrete human experiences and is rather about the history of consciousness, not about psychological development. Stanley Cavell offers a more psychological, yet philosophically grounded, account of the risks of avoidance and the power of acknowledgement. See Cavell 1979.

29. Terr 1990.

30. Not only Holocaust victims, but other survivors of trauma, including rape victims, repeatedly describe the numbing confusion and apathy they experience when others cannot genuinely recognize their suffering. Brison 1996, p. 29.

31. Many survivors married other survivors whom they met after they left the camps. Many of these couples did not discuss their traumatic experiences but sought partners who could understand without explanation. Survivors were often silent about their experiences with their own children, although they closely affiliated with other survivors in formal and informal social groups throughout their lives. Atina Grossman, personal communication, January 1998.

32. "Rape survivors, who typically have difficulty getting angry with their assailants, find that they are able to get angry on their own behalf by first getting angry on behalf of others. . . . [This] suggests that healing from trauma takes place through a kind of splitting off of the traumatized self, with which one is then able to empathize, just as one empathizes with others. The loss of a trauma survivor's former self is typically described by analogy to the loss of a beloved other. And yet, in grieving for another, one often says, 'its as though a part of myself has died.' It is not clear whether this circular comparison is a case of language failing us or, on the contrary, revealing a deep truth about selfhood and connectedness. But the essential point is that, by finding (some aspects of) one's lost self in another person, one can manage (to a greater or lesser degree) to reconnect with it and to reintegrate one's various selves into a coherent personality." Brison, p. 30, referring also to Koss and Harvey 1991.

33. Kant 1964, p. 430.

34. Korsgaard, p. 196.

35. Herman 1993a.

36. For a classic psychoanalytic article on this, see Strachey 1981 (1934).

37. Arthur Kleinman sees such questions as the bedrock of patient-centered care. Kleinman 1988.

38. Notably, the view of life as a project requiring sustaining or generating meaning in an ongoing way is distinctively existential and nowhere to be found in Kantian conceptions of autonomy. Further, speaking of *individual* life projects makes philosophical assumptions that are currently being questioned regarding personal identity and authenticity.

39. See Cassel 1982.

40. Gawande 1999.

41. Cassell and Quill 1996.

SIX

Cultivating Empathy in Medical Practice

Despite using a rhetoric of detachment, doctors do empathize with patients. However, they also sympathize with, over-identify with, take a detached knowing stance towards, and otherwise react to patients in ways that have been conflated with empathy. The benefit of the model of empathy as emotion-guided imagining developed here is that it permits a focus on developing some specific skills, rather than simply exhorting physicians to have compassion. At the same time, conceptualizing empathy as involving emotional engagement permits examining those aspects of medical training that impair emotional engagement. Although this book does not specifically address the ways by which physicians are socialized to detach, much work has been done in this area. Further, the recent emphasis on training physicians for empathy has brought with it some serious attempts to change the basic conditions that lead physicians to emotional disengagement, such as providing an emotionally supportive introduction early in medical training to such difficult experiences as dissecting cadavers.[1]

From Certainty to Curiosity

One key path to cultivating empathy is to help students develop and retain their engaged curiosity about other people's distinct experiences. A sense of knowing too much too soon about patients will impede this process. This openness is very difficult for doctors to achieve, given the time pressures of medical practice, the need for rapid diagnoses, and the pressure on physicians to know rather than to express uncertainty.[2]

Yet great power resides in not knowing too soon and in being genuinely curious about patients' views. Curiosity requires suspending judgment and allowing oneself to be uncertain. As such, it directs empathy toward ongoing discovery, rather than fixing the physician upon any one way of imagining another's feelings. The curiosity inducive to empathy is of a particular kind and can be distinguished from prurience and obsessive interest in details. This curiosity is grounded in an affective experience of connecting—wanting to relate to another person as another self, as a center of meaning and initiative. Rather than exhorting physicians to have extraordinary concern for their patients, empathy is promoted by cultivating the "natural" curiosity about other people's perspectives that motivates sociality and friendship. This is not to say that doctors simply use natural curiosity without contrivance. Continual openness towards strangers, including people one might not like, is a learned skill, but one that capitalizes on pre-existing curiosity.

Fortunately, although a physician cannot directly will herself to empathize, by cultivating curiosity she can *develop* empathy. For example, an attending physician, Sheldon Margen, noticed that his ambitious medical residents tended to give short shrift on rounds to older stroke patients, referring to them as "crocks," seeing their diseases as uninteresting. He designated every Friday as a time for each resident to spend an hour gathering a personal history from a patient with a known medical diagnosis. Despite initial resistance, the residents found themselves developing empathy for these patients, who told them detailed stories about their illness and life experiences. When one person actually listens to another person's story, emotional resonance and empathy often occur effortlessly. In *The Healer's Power* physician-scholar Howard Brody originated the phrase "empathic curiosity" to describe this link.[3]

Even during brief office visits, patients telling their stories can elicit empathy in physicians unless other stresses or barriers prohibit emotional engagement. One approach to teaching empathy, inspired by Rita Charon and others teaching in medical schools, is to have medical students write, in addition to the typical medical history, a narrative of the illness from the patient's perspective.[4] Charon has also worked with physicians by having them write narratives of their most troubling encounters with patients. The physicians felt that such practices build empathy and an awareness of ethical complexity.[5]

Part of what I mean by the term *curiosity* is ongoing attentiveness and openness to what patients communicate, verbally and nonverbally. In contrast to the detached insight model, which emphasizes the physician's preexisting knowledge of typical emotions, the model of empathy developed here emphasizes associating together, a process of communication. An important corrective to the risk of being too knowing is to adhere to using the patient's own words and image-laden stories. Mr. Smith bitterly said treatment was "useless, a waste." Ms. G. said that asking her to talk about her thoughts was "the cruelest thing anyone has ever done to me." These powerful words needed to be repeated to make specific communication about the patient's experience possible. Although empathy is not reducible to a kind of mechanistic "mirroring," patients who feel that their doctors pay careful attention are more likely to talk about their situations, and listening to patients tell their stories in their own words helps engender empathy.

Developing awareness of nonverbal as well as verbal cues helps promote empathy. It is well established that people communicate a great deal of information almost instantaneously through body language, vocal tone, and other pre-reflective cues.[6] Recent research has examined how, in the medical setting, empathy involves capitalizing on such cues. In a study cited earlier from the *Journal of the American Medical Association*, researchers closely observed patient–physician interactions and noted that before patients talked about aspects of their history that were emotional, they gave hints, often through gestures.[7] When physicians responded to these cues in a detached manner, no disclosure took place. In contrast, when physicians showed that they were affectively engaged at such moments, patients talked about emotionally laden aspects of their illnesses and lives, giving fuller histories.[8]

This study provides empirical support for the model of empathy developed in this book, with its emphasis on spontaneous resonance and nonverbal attunement to others' moods. In contrast, modeling empathy as detached insight does not guide physicians to develop the kind of nonverbal attunement that seems so essential in clinical settings. Further, as this empirical study describes, empathic physicians are affectively guided in an ongoing way that shapes the timing of their questions and silences.

This coheres with the model of empathy as affect-guided imagining, because it requires that affects guide, rather than merely trigger, empathy.

However, encouraging physicians to read nonverbal messages creates real risks of projection and other errors. Psychological and social differences preclude a universal way of translating gestures. For example, a stoic patient's curved lips may be a grimace hiding pain rather than a smile indicating that all is well. Gestures are multivalent and can cause verbal and nonverbal messages to be at odds, as when a patient says everything is fine while wringing her hands. Further, studies show that people are, overall, greatly biased by their initial affective reactions to nonverbal communication and make unwarranted judgments about a person's character after mere seconds of observation.[9] To avoid such unwarranted judgments, physicians might seek to put their reading of patients' nonverbal messages into words, just as they repeat important phrases, to elicit patients' critical appraisals and elaborations. Yet sometimes interpreting a patient's gestures can make her feel ashamed or anxious, rather than understood. For example, the hand-wringing woman who says she is fine might have some important psychological reason to keep her worry out of consciousness.[10] For all these reasons, physicians need to pay attention to nonverbal interactions as important clues warranting further inquiry, but to avoid presumptions about the patient's state of mind.

Another important use of curiosity is to prevent physicians from conflating intense resonance feelings with an accurate understanding of a patient's distinct situation. Without ongoing curiosity, a physician can make the mistake of thinking that the intensity of her own affective experience corresponds to the accuracy or depth of her understanding of a patient. Recall that I argued in chapter 4 that empathy cannot be merely a matter of entertaining hypotheses about another, but rather must involve having an experience of the other's emotions as present and real. Resonating, however, can mislead doctors into thinking that they are penetrating to the core of a patient's character. However, all that moments of empathy ever yield is an imagined portrayal of another person's existing emotion, that is, her state of mind at *one point in time*. No person in any state of mind has direct access to his own, or anyone else's, overall emotional character and motives.[11] Empathy, therefore, does not supplant other forms of psychological inquiry.

Nor does it supplant learning about cultural differences. Throughout this book I have spoken of patients and doctors as dyads, an abstraction that de-emphasizes the influences of culture, power, and the structure of medical practice. However, I do not mean to suggest that empathy operates independently of these factors. The structure of medical practice raises critical issues of power and voice, and cultural, gender, and other differences deeply influence medical care. Empathy is embedded in these social interactions, and differences in language, style, and values influence empathy. Therefore, issues of cultural difference, sensitivity, identification, and devaluing need to be reflectively addressed in educating physicians about empathy.[12]

Status, race, and gender differences influence patient–physician communication. Unrecognized, such differences can lead to serious consequences. For example, in a study of patients with lung cancer who were eligible for experimental surgery, black patients who held the same insurance and who were of the same socioeconomic and health status as white patients received less surgery, resulting in lower survival rates.[13] One hypothesis raised by these findings is that white physicians may not have understood the perspectives of black patients. Black patients may have found white physicians offering them unproven, or experimental, cancer treatments particularly untrustworthy, given the legacy of Tuskegee and other uses of disadvantaged blacks as research subjects. In such cases, white physicians may have failed black patients by not addressing the meaning the treatment might have for the patient, leading to more treatment refusals.

This example and others like it do not indicate, in my view, that white physicians are fundamentally incapable of empathizing with black patients' concerns, but rather the need for vigilance about cultural and other differences and about the distinct meanings of medical treatments for patients and doctors. Empathy does not, in and of itself, bridge divides created by cultural ignorance. Sensitizing physicians to both their own prejudices as well as the societal and cultural influences implicated in medical decisions is crucial.

Training physicians to be curious about patients' distinct worlds is critical for integrating empathy into medicine. This can serve as a corrective to physicians presuming to know aspects of their patients' experiences that they do not know. One area in which this is especially needed is in treating people with disabilities. An unfortunate research finding is that physicians treat patients with cognitive disabilities with inadequate understanding and respect.[14] A similar record of failures applies to caring for patients with physical disabilities. Apparently, disabled patients are routinely perceived as "other" by physicians, a perception that denies the spectrum of disabilities, visible or not, experienced by patients and by physicians themselves.[15] Crucial work to sensitize physicians to living with disabilities is under way.[16]

Yet even under the best of circumstances, an able-bodied physician's empathy may be helpful but not sufficient for establishing a common experiential "world" with patients with disabilities and other life experiences that individual physicians have not had. A physician needs to learn the limits of empathy and to recognize when he is not adequately grasping a patient's experience. Even though empathy extends a person's understanding of illness beyond her own direct experience, this extension may not involve a full comprehension of what illness and disability involve. My imagining of Mr. Smith's position seems to correspond to this. Having a mobile body, I could not fully imagine either his paralysis or his precise sense of frustration at his immobility, which was not merely the summation of physical paralysis and emotional hopelessness, but a holistic experience of feeling trapped.[17]

It is critical for physicians to recognize those aspects of their patients' experiences of disabilities that they cannot adequately imagine and to find other sources of support for such patients. For example, a nineteen-year-old athletic college student with severe Crohn's disease was so depressed about pending surgery that would leave him with a colostomy that he refused the surgery, despite a high risk of mortality without it. He said that he could not enjoy a life without competitive sports, and when his doctors tried to describe alternative physical options, they met with little success. One young male resident took extra time to speak with him and came to understand that it was upsetting for the patient to speak with this doctor about what he most feared, the loss of his sense of virility and sexuality, which this doctor exuded. The doctor asked the patient to meet with a nurse, a woman in her thirties who had a colostomy. She described to him her own experience as a sexual person with a colostomy, and through their meeting the young man was left with hope about a sex life after the surgery.

What role did empathy play in this intervention? It is not clear from this vignette whether the therapeutic influence of the nurse resulted from her empathy for this patient's individual perspective or from her providing an inspiring example. It is probable that both occurred. Because empathy depends on imagining what, concretely, another person is experiencing, it makes sense that it can be enhanced when one knows more about what an illness or treatment is like. However, a physician's having a medical problem similar to his patient's does not automatically or necessarily facilitate empathy. For one thing, the risks of over-identification and projection are great when people face similar illnesses, or even similar risk factors. On the other hand, this nurse demonstrated the possibility of living fully with a disability, and this might have instilled hope, independently of any empathic communication that occurred. This indicates that empathy is not the only way to make emotional contact in a therapeutic way.

In this case, I believe the resident physician represented a model for integrating empathy into medical care. Although the patient spoke to others only of his interest in sports, he felt sufficiently heard to tell the resident about his fears regarding his sexuality. Yet, the patient found it difficult to hear anything reassuring that this young male physician might say. The resident doctor recognized that no words coming from him could provide reassurance because the patient felt too threatened. Appreciating the patient's subjective view, he called in someone whom he hoped the patient would not find threatening and might find reassuring. By decentering from his own point of view and imagining how the patient felt, the resident helped in a way that using his own authority to reassure the patient would not have accomplished.

Notably, this case also illustrates how empathy works in a team setting. Because this book focuses on moments of physicians relating to patients, it may convey an inaccurate impression that empathy is not something that a team of caregivers can cultivate. Yet in practice nurses, social workers, and other caregivers are frequently sources of empathy. Integrating empathy into medicine means including it in the entire team's approach. However, doing this well requires that team members acknowledge their own uncertainties and limitations.

Teaching empathy, then, involves not only specific verbal and nonverbal skills, but also, and most importantly, a change in medical culture, from emphasizing premature knowing and certainty toward maintaining curiosity. Physicians who cultivate curiosity about others, sensitivity to their own emotional reactions, and an ongoing capacity to see the patient's situation, motives, and reactions as distinct from their own are likely to develop increasing empathic skills. The accuracy of empathy increases with effort. This does not preclude the occurrence of sudden, deeply accurate empathic insights about a person. These insights may be greatly facilitated by prior reflective thought about the other person. That is, such moments may be like the flashes of discovery one has after long periods of working through one's ideas. On the other hand, physicians often come to understand patients deeply through empathic communication, without such flashes ever occurring.[18]

Emotional Irrationality Revisited: Finding the Therapeutic Opportunity

A gap remains in this book, which began by focusing on failed patient–physician communication in a setting of intense emotional irrationality and then described how physicians can harness ordinary emotional reasoning to cultivate empathy. A remaining question is what doctors are supposed to do when they find themselves caught emotionally in the "morass of the patient's problems" (which Aring warned all doctors to avoid). In this section I take a final, controversial step, which is to argue that far from avoiding feeling disturbed by their patients' suffering, physicians might welcome these moments. The instances in which a patient's feelings of helplessness and fear induce similar feelings in her physician offer unique therapeutic opportunities.

I propose at least two reasons that those moments in which doctors are deeply affected by patients are unique opportunities for empathy. First, patients are often unaware of their own intolerable emotional states and reveal few clues to those states, except those that arise because of the impact they have on other people. In such cases, the doctor's own reactions to the patient are necessary clues to the patient's otherwise hidden emotional experience.

Second, moments of unconscious emotional communication are those in which patients are most open to physicians' influence, be it destructive or therapeutic. It is unlikely that at such moments doctors can bypass these possibilities by detaching and maintaining a neutral emotional affect. When a patient is very frightened, a doctor's detachment might lead the patient to believe that the doctor does not understand her emotional predicament or does not care what happens to her. Doctors believe that by detaching and reviewing the problems logically, they can persuade patients to be more rational. But for a patient in the throes of emotional irrationality, all cognitive input, including excellent logical arguments, is easily distorted.

For example, the mother of a ten-year-old boy with severe Tourette's syndrome felt terribly anxious after seeing her child's psychiatrist, who recommended antipsychotic medication for her son. The physician was so calm and unemotional that she felt that he was minimizing the health threat and stigma that such medication brought to her mind, and she decided she could not trust him. The psychiatrist learned that for some patients, his neutral style, which he had cultivated deliberately to calm patients and help them think more clearly, was having the opposite effect.[19]

The point of this vignette is that diverse patients need different things from physicians to process difficult news. The detached physician projects calmness and optimism and resists being moved inwardly. This paternal cultural icon has been held to with great tenacity, suggesting that great therapeutic power lies in a reassuring, confident professional stance. Yet, what is left out of this model is the need patients have first to make sure that the physician is sufficiently affected by their predicaments before relying on the physician's resilience and confidence.

Interestingly, Roter showed that of all the factors studied that were thought to affect patient trust, the most significant was the patient's perception that the doctor seem concerned or even worried about them. A doctor's apparent worry was much more likely to induce trust than cheerfulness or friendliness, which were expected to be more important.[20] This observation surprises us today, but perhaps it would not have surprised physicians from the Hippocratic era through the time of Hooker. They describe how the art of medicine involves allowing patients to create a host of sorrows that the physician feels and yet demonstrates can be handled with resiliency.

Why is it especially healing for patients to see that their physicians are *both* genuinely worried and otherwise emotionally moved by their predicaments *and* that they view their problems in a reassuring way? Throughout this book I have been developing the theme that emotional reasoning is an interpersonal process. This is of special importance when people are in irrational emotional states, because people rely on one another's capacities for emotional reasoning to overcome such irrationality. This is simply the positive side of the interaction that occurred in Ms. G.'s case, when her physicians' inability to process her intense emotions exacerbated her concretized emotional states. What models do we have for the interpersonal processing of irrational emotions?

In the remainder of this chapter, I will suggest two distinct ways that physicians may help patients "work through" intense irrational emotions.[21] The first involves patients making use of physicians' capacities to reflect on emotions to regain their own mental freedom. The second, less cognitive account, involves patients experiencing their physicians as capable of withstanding emotional impact from them, and yet not abandoning them.

Regaining Mental Freedom

Let me return to the discussion begun in chapter 4 about how an empathic listener may help a person in a catastrophic emotional state regain mental freedom. How is empathy effective? Part of a patient's recognizing that a doctor is genuinely grasping his situation empathically involves imagining how the doctor sees his subjective experience. For example, when Mr. Smith recognized my empathy, he saw that I grasped his enormous anger at being treated with no respect for his dignity. He saw that I imagined him as a powerful person and hence felt that I respected him. In contrast, when I simply felt sorry for him at the beginning, seeing his paralyzed body, he knew that I saw him then as merely pitiable.

For the patient to absorb the doctor's thinking regarding his emotional predicament requires mental processes that are similar to the doctor's imagining how the patient feels. However, rather than the physician imaginatively "imitating," or taking on, the patient's emotions, the patient is imaginatively "imitating," or taking on, the physician's *interpretation* of her emotional predicament.

My hypothesis about the therapeutic mechanism of projective identification transformed into empathy is as follows. When a person recognizes that another is both experiencing, and yet not fully in the grips of, her catastrophic mental state, she can recognize that she herself is *holding* a particular emotional perspective. This recognition disrupts her from attributing her view to external, concrete reality. When a depressed patient feels that her physician empathically grasps the bleakness of her perceived future, but that physician does not believe that her future really is so hopeless, she might begin to see that she is subject to a depressed state of mind.

One model for how empathy can be transformative in this way comes from a philosophical analysis of how people overcome compartmentalization of their mental states. Donald Davidson and Marcia Cavell developed this model to explain self-deception. They describe how people can fool themselves into maintaining irrational beliefs by compartmentalizing these views into separate spheres of mental life that are not accountable to one another.

Insofar as an attitude remains compartmentalized, it can act persuasively, influencing other attitudes, without having to meet any standard of internal coherence or reasonableness. Ms. G. blocked out awareness that she *held* a belief about her future and acted as if it were an external fact that her future was hopeless. This belief thus constantly influenced her without being challenged by any other thoughts or observations. In contrast, consciously to acknowledge that one is holding a belief, according to Davidson, forces one to differentiate it from other beliefs and to relate it to these other beliefs.

Corresponding to this philosophical model, psychoanalytic models have been proposed of how a person develops the capacity to think about overwhelming emotions with another person's help. These models usually refer to infancy and are therefore not intended to apply concretely to the circumstances of adult patients and physicians. A key psychoanalytic theory of how infants learn to manage irrational emotions comes from Wilfred Bion.[22]

Bion emphasizes that when an infant "projects" distress into the mother, this distress must genuinely be felt by the mother for her mental processes to be a positive influence. Ideally, she can feel the distress, but also think about this distress and convey to the baby that she understands the severity but also will alleviate the discomfort. The key similarity between Davidson's and Bion's accounts is that another sees (in Bion's case, empathizes with) the distress, yet is able to manipulate it flexibly as a state of mind, and this engenders a capacity to stand apart from an overwhelming state of mind in the sufferer.

Alternatively, Bion argues, if the mother cannot respond with both empathy and the capacity to think and solve problems, the baby not only grows more intensely distressed, but the projective processes become concretized. For example, if the mother is indifferent or becomes very upset, the baby may develop a sense that the world *is* distressing, that something terrible *will* happen. He is not "thinking," in the sense of flexibly interacting with the mother to gain reassurance, but rather forming a sense of conviction or a concretized reality.

How does all this apply to the clinical setting? An adult facing serious threats or losses needs to bear what feels intolerable and to regenerate a sense of safety. If we now envision an adult patient, Ms. G., for example, in a concretized state of fear, we can consider various ways that her projections served as archaic communications to her physicians and various ways that they could have responded that would have been useful to her. Her doctors did not empathically hold her view of the future in mind and think about it simultaneously. In the absence of this, Ms. G.'s catastrophic thinking "hardened," and she developed a conviction that she knew the future. If, instead, they had been able to receive her emotional message, her "projected" terror, and simultaneously think about it, perhaps she, too, could have regained the capacity to think more flexibly. Note that what makes projective identification potentially therapeutic is precisely the empathic, not sympathetic or detached, reception of the projection.

My hypothesis is that when someone who is subject to an irrational concretized emotion recognizes that a trusted other sees her as subject to a particular state of mind, she may be able to recognize that she is subject to a point of view. We might say that another person's assumption of Ms. G.'s emotional view while differentiating it as a point of view could be a vehicle for Ms. G. to do the same. The moment such complex recognition took place, Ms. G.'s concretized belief might lose its isolation from her other beliefs and might then become something she could cognitively as well as affectively "work through."[23] Once people associate together, an internal pressure builds toward challenging the absoluteness, or certainty, of their emotional convictions. The matter being empathized about is, as it were, forced to be accountable to a norm of realism, aptness, and accuracy.

There are other ways in which recognizing that one is subject to a state of mind can be therapeutic. One grasps that this state of mind can pass into other states of mind (the definition of a state). This awareness, in and of itself, makes it possible to think about or become curious about one's view. It is akin to recognizing that one is subject to a certain visual perspective. Recognizing that one is experiencing from a particular perspective allows one to question whether alternative perspectives on the matter might exist and also to inquire into the intrapsychic basis of one's own perspective.

Thus, we have come full circle from the model of empathy as the doctor projecting his or her personality into the patient to one in which empathy involves the doctor accepting and consciously experiencing the patient's projections. Receiving patients' projections while being able to think openly about the experiences is a crucial way for doctors to empathize with patients in difficult emotional states.[24]

Non-Abandonment

Research shows that even years after receiving a diagnosis of cancer, patients and their families report being seriously affected by their physicians' method of communication. Patients describe doctors telling them too much all at once and then leaving them unaided in thinking about what was said. People specifically report as harmful not the information overload, per se, but the sense that the doctor wanted to dump the information in a blunt, factual way, rather than struggle emotionally with the patient. The patients especially felt that they needed their doctors to help them emotionally digest the information to make it tolerable.[25] They noted that their doctors did not seem cruel, but that they felt abandoned by them. Combining this research with several other studies suggests that what makes such diagnoses tolerable is less a cognitive matter and more a matter of the physician's emotional engagement. In response to the research on cancer patients and their families, educators are training physicians to accept and convey emotional messages when giving bad news.[26,27]

The example of hearing a cancer diagnosis brings up, again, the centrality of grieving to healing. As mentioned earlier, grieving is a multifaceted process in which people are transiently preoccupied with irrational emotions, including denial, bargaining to reverse the loss, and rage at the universe for singling them out.[28] People need to go through these irrational emotional states before they come to a fuller acceptance of their losses.

Why is it so challenging for physicians to provide the support patients need to progress through these phases toward recovery? Although, as already mentioned, some of the problem may be the physicians' own fears of death and dying and the severe time constraints of current medical practice, another important issue is at stake. When patients are subject to intense, irrational emotions, they may not engage directly in telling about their needs, but more often show them by having an emotional impact (usually negative) on their medical team. Physicians need special skills to transform the negative emotional projections they experience into therapeutic opportunities.

Donald Winnicott, a psychoanalyst and pediatrician, emphasizes how valuable it is for a caregiver to receive negative projected emotions to help others process their emotions. He describes how rage, denial, and other troubling attitudes that may erupt between patients and their physicians can be accepted and acknowledged by physicians in ways that may facilitate patients in making fuller emotional recoveries.[29] When a suffering person feels that another person is affected by her grief, sense of catastrophe, or fear, and yet remains vital and emotionally present, this helps her retain her own sense of vitality.[30]

Winnicott's model is largely spelled out in terms of early development, (infants with mothers), and thus, unfortunately, risks bringing to mind infantilizing views of patients. However, his ideas about projection and empathy have been developed for many adult models that imply no inequality.[31] According to Winnicott, a mother's capacity to feel an infant's pain, yet not be destroyed by it, allows the infant to establish a belief in resilient others outside his control.[32] The result of this "good-enough," or nonretaliatory, mothering is that the child can experience a "continuity of being," a feeling of "aliveness" or interest in life. Winnicott describes how this sense of continuity of being, of a personal psychic reality, helps people face loss throughout life and regenerate a sense of security and ongoingness.[33] During illness in adult life, a need exists to draw from this more basic sense of ongoingness. When a person faces a serious threat to his future he feels impotent. He may begin to regain a sense of potency through an interpersonal struggle of the sort Winnicott describes.

Recall that Ms. G. became enraged with me, telling me that I had hurt her like no one else ever had. Her intense anger resembled the kind of desperately hurt rage one would expect she might feel toward her husband but was not yet ready to face. A psychiatrist who specializes in helping people after trauma describes such moments as the essential therapeutic moment: patients begin to experience their intolerable affects, but toward the therapist, whose capacity to feel and endure the communicated affect helps the patient bear it.[34] Perhaps, if Ms. G. and I had had a few more days to meet and she had continued to express this anger while finding that I did not abandon her, she might have come to view her own mental states as less threatening. Winnicott specifically says that when accompanied in this way, a distressed person may regain the capacity to be "alone," which is akin to what was described in chapter 5 as being able to wander inside one's own imagination.[35]

Winnicott further offers a way for doctors to respond therapeutically rather than destructively to patients whom they find frustrating or even threatening. Before Mr. Smith raged at me, he vented anger toward his other doctors and nurses, and they either reacted with false neutrality, making him feel patronized, or avoided him altogether. Simply by staying emotionally attuned and withstanding all impulses to flee during my second visit to him (recall that I did flee at the end of the first meeting), a therapeutic encounter became possible. It was when he began yelling at me that he connected with me for the first time.

When patients feel extremely vulnerable, attempts to provoke their doctors may be attempts to intuit indestructability. From this perspective, doctors always have something to offer patients in emotional distress: their own "nonretaliatory durability." Sometimes, demonstrating this characteristic involves very concrete steps. For example, insofar as doctors inadvertently avoid spending time seeing patients who engender feelings of anger or hopelessness in them, awareness of these emotional tendencies can lead to consciously reversing such practices. Deliberately making daily visits that the patient can count on, at a consistent time and for a consistent duration, can have a positive impact.

Winnicott's emphasis on *accompanying* the suffering patient thus provides a model that extends beyond Bion's mentalistic account in guiding physicians to respond therapeutically to patients' rage, anxiety, and other difficult emotions. In addition, this model is helpful for treating patients who refuse to communicate. Ironically, in a book about empathic communication, the cases that emerged as central involved patients at moments when they refused to communicate, Ms. G. and Mr. Smith. How can physicians stay emotionally engaged with patients who refuse communication?

Safeguarding some aspect of the self from overt communication while still feeling accompanied can be fundamental to feeling real. A literary example, Tolstoy's *The Death of Ivan Illych*, illustrates this approach. Illych, like Ms. G., is dying in excruciating pain. Screaming for days, he is pained less by his physical condition than by the coinciding recognition of the falsity of his longstanding relationships. His servant, Gerasim, stays with him at night, holding his legs to alleviate his pain, but also witnessing his suffering nonjudgmentally. To his astonishment, Illych finds in this simple companionship the alleviation of his suffering, yet it inspires him, not to communicate, but to withdraw into his own being and die his own death. His last act is to refuse to occupy his social persona, saying only "I won't." Yet, in so doing, he regains a feeling of being real that had eluded him since early childhood.[36]

The link between refusing to communicate, the capacity to experience being in one's aloneness, and the need for accompaniment and empathy has been articulated by Winnicott. I adapt his warning (written for psychiatrists) for all physicians as a final attempt to redress what went wrong in Ms. G.'s case, and as a balance to this book's emphasis on articulating meaning and promoting autonomy. The warning goes something like this: It takes time for patients to seek self-awareness, and, even so, some aspects of the self are permanently safeguarded by resisting communication. Physicians are increasingly under pressure to rush patients through medical decision making. Rushing creates the risk that patients will merely comply with, instead of participate in, treatment decisions, as well as the risk that patients will not feel real and authentic. Ms. G. and others in catastrophic states often feel so fragmented or shocked by their circumstances that they desperately need to regain a sense of "feeling real."[37] To ask a patient, as I did Ms. G., to put her suffering into words is to ask her to deliver it over to others, to what Winnicott calls the "not-me." He sees a pitfall in rushing patients to articulate, rather than waiting patiently while accompanying the patient: "We [healers] suddenly become not-me for the patient, and then we know too much, and we are dangerous because we are too nearly in communication with the central still and silent spot of the patient's ego-organization."[38] Perhaps for Ms. G., allowing her to withdraw into a restorative experience of aloneness while staying emotionally present would have been therapeutic, even if the only benefit of this had been that she died in the hospital accompanied rather than alone.

The idea that accompanying patients in their suffering can be therapeutic leads to an alternative to the ideal of detached concern for patient–physician interactions. The visual metaphor of the "objective" doctor standing before the patient and "seeing through" her irrational emotions ought to be replaced with a paradigm in which the patient "makes use of" the doctor's nonretaliatory emotional presence to go through the necessarily irrational emotional phases of grieving. This model would make it possible to transform how doctors respond to patients like Ms. G., whose certainty that her future was hopeless should trigger reflection and empathy.

Medical practice involves more than mending physical bodies: it involves healing emotional states, but the challenge to discern where emotional healing is needed is a formidable one, even in ordinary medical encounters. Emotional receptivity is needed if physicians are to acknowledge the pain and suffering that patients do not, and sometimes cannot, put into words. This is because suffering is, by definition, difficult to bear, and thus is denied, resisted, hidden, or otherwise kept out of awareness.

Discerning the core of suffering is an uphill battle against the defenses we all have against dying, loss, abandonment, shame, and self-fragmentation. Intense states of suffering that involve fragmentation of the self are communicated nonverbally, primarily through inducing affective states in others.[39] By enduring with patients emotionally, physicians can help alleviate suffering that cannot be fully translated into words. By allowing patients to move them emotionally, it is as if physicians allow patients to *inscribe* in them, or use them to contain, what is otherwise intolerable to hold onto and "work through."

William Carlos Williams describes his own struggles to stay open emotionally while caring for patients. When he became coarse and numb, his patients helped him return to his own humanity. The physician and writer Robert Coles describes such moments as the epiphanies that enrich medical practice, when the real meaning of medical treatment is suddenly illuminated in terms of hidden personal meanings.[40] A physician who allows his patients to move him emotionally will enrich his own experience of doctoring.

The irony of detachment is that in seeking "objective reality," physicians ignore an important source of understanding reality. Through empathy, physicians allow patients' suffering and emotional needs to be real. Ultimately, physicians and patients need each other to face illness in a humane way. By allowing patients to move them emotionally, physicians enable more than the physical repair of bodies; they allow healing to begin.

NOTES

1. For example, Thomas Cole at the University of Texas made a film about gross anatomy lab, that humanizes the people who donate their bodies.

2. A classic study of physician attitudes toward uncertainty is *Experiment Perilous*, Fox 1998. A more recent one is Kvale et al. 1999.

3. On the relationship between curiosity and resonance in empathy see Halpern 1993. See also Howard Brody on empathic curiosity, 1992.

4. Charon 1993. In the same collected volume, Howard Spiro emphasizes the use of narratives in teaching empathy on ward rounds. See Spiro 1993.

5. Charon 1996 and Charon 1995.

6. Gladwell 2000.

7. Suchman et al. 1997.

8. *Ibid.*

9. Gladwell 2000.

10. Further, physicians also communicate through gestures that influence patients' gestures, yet physicians are often unconscious of this dialogue. See Sullivan 1953.

11. Recall from chapter 4 Tugendhat's and Stein's argument against special knowledge of our motives and character through direct introspection. That is, they argue that we come to know our motives as we come to know other people's motives, by experiencing ourselves as social agents over time.

12. Also see Lipsyte 1998.

13. Bach et al. 1999.

14. French 1996.

15. See, for example, Murphy 1990.

16. French 1996.

17. I am indebted to Patricia Benner for emphasizing this point.

18. See Buie 1981, Berger 1984, Berger 1987, and Basch 1983.

19. Personal communication, Dr. Russell Rief, a pediatrician, September 1999.

20. Roter et al. 1998.

21. I use the phrase *working through* to refer to processing emotions both affectively and cognitively, resulting in the ability to see things with greater flexibility. This use is influenced by the psychoanalytic concept of working through. See "Remembering, Repeating and Working Through" in Freud 1966, v. 12, pp. 147–156.

22. Bion argues that a parent's tolerance of projected emotions from a child helps develop the child's capacity to think through her own emotions. His essay, "On Thinking," describes how children's projective identifications with their parents create a direct opportunity for them to take in their parents' emotional capacities, for better or worse. Projective identification, Bion argues, is a primary way that infants communicate with their mothers. If, for example, an infant is hungry and starts to cry, this action distresses the mother. The infant can then observe the mother's discomfort as it is "projected" outward and identify with the mother's distress. See Bion 1962.

23. Freud 1966.

24. Under such favorable circumstances, the phrases *projective identification* and *empathy* are describing a single temporal event from two different perspectives. The emphasis on identification accentuates the fact that the patient identifies with her own emotions projected into the doctor.

25. See, for example, Campbell and Sanson-Fisher 1998; Girgis and Sanson-Fisher 1998; Ptacek and Eberhardt 1996; Walsh, Girgis, and Sanson-Fisher 1998; and Girgis and Sanson-Fisher 1995.

26. These articles report on an innovative program for training physicians to be emotionally attuned when giving prognostic information to cancer patients. See Ptacek and Eberhardt 1996 and Ptacek et al. 1999.

27. Pediatrician Jody Heyman describes how physicians help not only patients, but their families, by simply staying with them when they cry or otherwise express their grief

over a dying child, rather than leaving the room immediately, as doctors often do. See Heymann 1995.

28. Although Kübler-Ross, who described these stages, has been criticized for claiming that they occur in a neat progression, her description of such irrational states is consistent with earlier work by Bowlby, ongoing work of anthropologists in other cultures, and the clinical experiences of many patients, family members, and physicians. See Kübler-Ross 1969.

29. Winnicott 1949a.

30. Winnicott describes how children faced with loss are preoccupied with games of finding and losing, and destroying and restoring transitional objects, such as teddy bears and blankets. His hypothesis is that a child "destroys" an object because he has begun to experience it as separate and outside his subjective control; the child "places" the object outside his omnipotent control because he is aware of having destroyed it. Thus the child "uses" and "destroys" the object because it has become real, and the object becomes real because it has been "used" and "destroyed. The fact that the object withstands the child's destructive feelings is the crucial point. Greenberg and Mitchell 1983, p. 196.

31. See, for example, the couples therapy literature showing how partners project in order to convey messages to each other. See Doane and Diamone 1994.

32. The surviving object is a metaphor for, or representative of, the mother's "nonretaliatory durability." (Winnicott's focus is on the mother, but by using his language I do not mean to exclude a father or other caregiver's capacity to play this role.) A famous quote of Winnicott's is that there are no "infants" alone, only "infants with mothers," by which he means that people develop their sense of themselves in constant interaction with their caregivers. See also Greenberg and Mitchell, 1983, p. 196.

33. See "Ego Distortions in Terms of True and False Self" in Winnicott 1965.

34. Robert Pynoos, personal communication, May 2000.

35. The paradox of being in oneself free of social concerns, and yet of being accompanied and not abandoned, is explored in the essay "The Capacity to Be Alone" in Winnicott 1965.

36. Tolstoy 1981.

37. Brison 1996, pp. 30–31.

38. Winnicott 1965, p. 189.

39. Elaine Scarry writes about how extreme states of suffering can never be adequately verbally described. See Scarry 1993.

40. Coles 1989, pp. 117–118.

Bibliography

Alford, B. A., and A. T. Beck. 1997. Therapeutic interpersonal support in cognitive therapy. *Journal of Psychotherapy Integration* 7(2):105–117.

Angell, M. 1993. The doctor as double agent. *The Kennedy Institute of Ethics Journal* (September):279–286.

Annas, G. J. 1984a. Elizabeth Bouvia: Whose space is this anyway? *Hastings Center Report* 16(2):24–25.

Annas, G. J. 1984b. When suicide prevention becomes brutality: The case of Elizabeth Bouvia. *Hastings Center Report* 14(2):20–22, 46.

Anstett, R. 1980. The difficult patient and the physician–patient relationship. *Journal of Family Practice* 11:281–286.

Appelbaum, P. S., C. W. Lidz, and A. Meisel. 1987. Patients who refuse treatment. In *Informed Consent: Legal Theory and Clinical Practice*, New York: Oxford University Press: 90–207.

Appelbaum, P. S., and L. H. Roth. 1982. *Treatment Refusal in Medical Hospitals*. Washington, DC: President's Commission for the Study of Ethical Problems in Medicine and Biomedical and Behavioral Research.

Aring, Charles. 1958. Sympathy and empathy. *Journal of the American Medical Association* 167(4):448–452.

Aristotle. 1988. *The Nicomachean Ethics*, edited by J. L. Ackrill and J. O. Urmson. Oxford: Oxford University Press.

Arnetz, B. B. 1997. Physicians' view of their work environment and organization. *Psychotherapy and Psychosomatics* 66(3):155–162.

Bach, P. B., et al. 1999. Racial differences in treatment of early-stage lung cancer. *New England Journal of Medicine* 341(16):1198–1231.

Balint, M. 1957. *The doctor, His Patient and the Illness*. New York: International Universities Press.

Barasch, M. 1998. *Modern Theories of Art*. Vol. 2. New York: New York University Press.

Barlow, D. H. 1988. *Anxiety and Its Disorders: The Nature and Treatment of Anxiety and Panic*. New York: Guilford Press.

Basch, M. 1983. Empathic understanding: A review of the concept and some theoretical considerations. *Journal of the American Psychoanalytic Assocation* 31:101–125.

Bates, D., ed. 1995. *Knowledge and the Scholarly Medical Traditions*. Cambridge: Cambridge University Press.

Baxter, L. 1992. Neuroimaging studies of obsessive compulsive disorder. *Psychiatric Clinics of North America* 15(4):871–884.

Beauchamp, T. L., and J. F. Childress. 1979. *Principles of Biomedical Ethics*. New York: Oxford University Press.

Beck, A. T. 1979. *Cognitive Therapy of Anxiety and Phobic Disorders*. Philadelphia: Center for Cognitive Therapy.

Belfiore, M. 1994. The group that takes care of itself: Art therapy to prevent burnout. *Arts in Psychotherapy* 21(2):119–126.

Benner, P., P. Hooper-Kyria Kidis, and D. Stannard. 1999. *Clinical Wisdom and Intervention in Critical Care*: A Thinking-in-Action Approach. Philadelphia: Saunders Press.

Berger, D. M. 1984. On the way to empathic understanding. *American Journal of Psychotherapy* (38):111–120.

Berger, D. M. 1987. *Clinical Empathy*. New Jersey: Jason Aronson.

Bertakis, K. D., D. Roter, and S. M. Putnam. 1991. The relationship of physician medical interview style to patient satisfaction. *Journal of Family Practice* 32(2): 175–181.

Bion, W. 1962. A theory of thinking. *International Journal of Psycho-analysis* 43(4,5):110–119.

Blanck, P. D., R. Rosenthal, and M. Vannicelli. 1986. Talking to and about patients: The therapist's tone of voice. In *Nonverbal Communication in the Clinical Context*, edited by P. D. Blanck, R. Buck, and R. Rosenthal. Univesity Park: Pennsylvania State University.

Bliss, M. 1999. *William Osler: A Life in Medicine*. Oxford: Oxford University Press.

Blumgart, H. 1964. Caring for the patient. *The New England Journal of Medicine* 270(9):449–456.

Bower, J. E., M. E. Kemeny, and S. E. Taylor. 1998. Cognitive processing, discovery of meaning, CD4 decline, and AIDS-related mortality among bereaved HIV-seropositive men. *Journal of Consulting and Clinical Psychology* 66(6):979–986.

Bowlby, J. 1982. Attachment and loss: Retrospect and prospect. *American Journal of Orthopsychiatry* 52(4):664–678.

Brison, S. J. 1996. Outliving oneself: Trauma, memory, and personal identity. In *Feminists Rethink the Self*, edited by D. Meyers. Boulder: Westview Press.

Brody, B. A. 1990. The role of philosophy in public policy and bioethics—introduction. *Journal of Medicine and Philosophy* 15(4):345–346.

Brody, H. 1992. *The Healer's Power*. New Haven: Yale University Press.

Buie, D. H. 1981. Empathy: Its nature and limitations. *Journal of the American Psychoanalytic Association* 29:281–307.

Cacioppo, J. T., and W. L. Gardner. 1999. Emotion. *Annual Review of Psychology* 50:191–214.

Calhoun, C. 1984. Cognitive emotions? In *What Is an Emotion?*, edited by C. Calhoun and R. C. Solomon. Oxford: Oxford University Press.

Campbell, E. M., and R. W. Sanson-Fisher. 1998. Breaking bad news 3: Encouraging the adoption of best practices. *Behavioral Medicine* 24 (Summer):73.

Casey, E. 1976. *Imaginings*. Bloomington: Indiana University Press.

Cassel, E. J. 1982. The nature of suffering and the goals of medicine. *New England Journal of Medicine* 306(11):639–645.

Castonguay, L. G. 1997. Support in psychotherapy: A common factor in need of empirical data, conceptual clarification, and clinical input. *Journal of Psychotherapy Integration* 7(2):99–117.

Cavell, M. 1998. Triangulation, one's own mind, and objectivity. *International Journal of Psycho-Analysis* 79(3):449–467.

Cavell, S. 1979. *The Claim of Reason*. New York: Oxford University Press.

Charon, R. 1993. The narrative road to empathy. In *Empathy and the Practice of Medicine*, edited by H. Spiro. New Haven: Yale University Press.

Charon, R., H. Brody, et.al. 1996. Literature and ethical medicine: Five cases from common practice. *Journal of Medicine and Philosophy* 21(3):243–265.

Charon, R., et.al. 1995. Literature and medicine: Contributions to clinical practice. *Annals of Internal Medicine* 122(8):599–606.

Christakis, N. A., and D. A. Asch. 1993. Biases in how physicians choose to withdraw life support. *Lancet* 342(8872):642–646.

Coles, R. 1989. *The Call of Stories*. Boston: Houghton Mifflin.

Cottle, M. 1999. Selling shyness: How doctors and drug companies created the "social phobia" epidemic. *The New Republic* 4(4,411):24–29.

Crutcher, J. E., and M. J. Bass. 1980. The difficult patient and the troubled physician. *Journal of Family Practice* 11:933–938.

Cushing, H. 1925. *The Life of Sir William Osler*. Oxford: Clarendon Press.

Damasio, A. 1994. *Descartes' Error: Emotion, Reason and the Human Brain*. New York: Grosset/Putnam.

Davidson, D. 1974. Paradoxes of irrationality. In *Freud: A Collection of Critical Essays*, edited by R. Wollheim. New York: Doubleday.

Deckard, G., et al. 1994. Physician burnout: An examination of personal, professional and organizational relationships. *Medical Care* 32(7):745–754.

Deigh, J. 1993. Cognitivism in the theory of emotions. *Ethics* 104:824–854.

Descartes, R. 1984. *Descartes: The Philosophical Works*. Translated by Haldane, E. and Ross, G. R. T. Edited by E. S. Haldane and G. R. T. Ross. New York: Cambridge University Press.

Descartes, R. 1970. *Descartes' Philosophical Letters*. Translated by A. Kenny. London: Oxford University Press.

De Sousa, R. 1987. *The Rationality of Emotions*. Boston: MIT Press.

Deutsch, H. 1970. Occult processes during psychoanalysis. In *Psychoanalysis and the Occult*, edited by G. Devereux. New York: International University Press.

Deyo, R. A., and A. K. Diehl. 1986. Patient satisfaction with medical care for low-back pain. *Spine* 11(1):28–30.

DiMatteo, M. R., A. Taranta, H. S. Friedman, and L. M. Prince. 1980. Predicting patient satisfaction from physician's nonverbal communication skills. *Medical Care* 18(4):376–387.

Doane, J., and D. Diamone. 1994. *Affect and Attachment in the Family*. New York: Basic Books.

Dossey, L. 1991. *Meaning and Medicine: Lessons from a Doctor's Tales of Breakthrough and Healing*. New York: Bantam Books.

Drane, J. F. 1985. The many faces of competency. *Hastings Center Report* 15(2):17–21.

Entralgo, P. L. 1969. *Doctor and Patient*. New York: MacGraw-Hill.

Farber, N. J., D. H. Novack, and M. K. O'Brien. 1997. Love, boundaries, and the patient–physician relationship. *Archives of Internal Medicine* 157(20):2291–2294.

Fawzy, F. I. 1995. A short term psycho-educational intervention for patients newly diagnosed melanoma. *Supportive Care in Cancer* 3(4):235–238.

Fawzy, F. I., and N. W. Fawzy. 1998. Group therapy in the cancer setting. *Journal of Psychosomatic Research* 45(3):191–200.

Fawzy, F. I., N. W. Fawzy, C. Hyun, R. Elashoff, D. Guthrie, J. L. Fahey, and D. L. Morton. 1993. Malignant melanoma: Effects of an early structured psychiatric intervention, coping, and affective state on recurrence and survival six years later. *Archives of General Psychiatry* 50:681–689.

Feldman, J. L., and B. J. Fitzpatrick. 1992. *Managed Mental Health Care: Administrative and Clinical Issues*. Washington, DC: American Psychiatric Press.

Fell, J. 1965. *Emotion in the Thought of Sartre*. New York: Columbia University Press.

Felman, S. 1987. *Jacques Lacan and the Adventure of Insight: Psychoanalysis in Contemporary Culture*. Cambridge, MA: Harvard University Press.

Fenichel, O. 1953. Identification. In *The Collected Papers of Otto Fenichel, First Series*. New York: Norton Publishers.

Fliess, R. 1942. The metapsychology of the analyst. *Psychoanalytic Quarterly* 11: 211–227.

Foucault, M. 1994. *The Birth of the Clinic: An Archaeology of Medical Perception*. Translated by A. M. Sheridan Smith. New York: Vintage Books.

Fox, R. C. 1998. *Experiment Perilous: Physicians and Patients Facing the Unknown*. Revised ed. New Brunswick, N.J.: Transaction Publishers.

Fox, R., and H. Lief. 1963. Training for "detached concern." In *The Psychological Basis of Medical Practice*, edited by H. Lief. New York: Harper & Row.

Frank, J., and J. Frank. 1991. *Healing and Persuasion: A Comparative Study of Psychotherapy*. 3rd ed. Baltimore: Johns Hopkins University Press.

Frankfurt, H. 1988. *The Importance of What We Care About*. New York: Cambridge University Press.

Frasure-Smith, N., F. Lesperance, and M. Talajic. 1995. The impact of negative emotions on prognosis following myocardial infarction: Is it more than depression? *Health Psychology* 14(5):388–398.

French, S. 1996. The attitudes of health professionals towards disabled people. In *Beyond Disability: Towards an Enabling Society*, edited by G. Hales et al. London: Sage Publications.

Freud, S. 1949. The external world. In *An Outline of Psychoanalysis*. New York: Norton.

Freud, S. 1959. *Group Psychology and Analysis of the Ego*. Translated by J. Strachey. New York: Norton.

Freud, S. 1966. *The Standard Edition of the Complete Works of Sigmund Freud (1953–74)*. Translated and edited by J. Strachey. 24 vols. London: Hogarth Press.

Gawande, A. 1999. Whose body is it anyway?: What doctors should do when patients make bad decisions. *The New Yorker*; 4 October 1999: 84–92.

Geskie, M. A., and J. Salasek. 1988. Attitudes of health care personnel towards persons with disabilities. In *Attitudes Towards Persons with Disabilities*, edited by H. Yuker. New York: Springer.

Girgis, A., and R. W. Sanson-Fisher. 1995. Breaking bad news: Consensus guidelines for medical practitioners. *Journal of Clinical Oncology* 13:2449–2456.

Girgis, A., and R. W. Sanson-Fisher. 1998. Breaking bad news 1: Current advice for clinicians. *Behavioral Medicine* 24(summer):53–59.

Gladwell, M. 2000. The new-boy network: What does a handshake mean? *The New Yorker*; 29 May 2000:68.

Glick, R., and S. Bone, eds. 1990. *Pleasure Beyond the Pleasure Principle: The Role of Affect in Motivation, Development and Adaptation*. New Haven, CT: Yale University Press.

Glick, S. M. 1997. Unlimited human autonomy—a cultural bias. *New England Journal of Medicine* 336(13):954–956.

Good, B. 1994. *Medicine, Rationality, and Experience: An Anthropological Perspective*. Edited by A. Carter. Cambridge: Cambridge University Press.

Good, M. J. D. 1991. The practice of biomedicine and the discourse on hope: A preliminary investigation into the culture of American oncology. In *Anthropologies of Medicine: A Colloquium on West European and North American perspectives*, edited by B. Pfleiderer and G. Bibeau. Braunschweig: F. Vieweg.

Good, M. J. D., B. J. Good, C. Schaffer, and S. E. Lind. 1990. American oncology and the discourse on hope. *Culture, Medicine and Psychiatry* 14:59–79.

Goodwin, J. M., J. S. Goodwin, and R. Kellner. 1979. Psychiatric symptoms in disliked medical patients. *Journal of the American Medical Association* 241(11): 1117–1120.

Gordon, D. 1988. Tenacious assumptions in western medicine. In *Biomedicine Examined*, edited by M. Lock and D. R. Gordon. Dordrecht: Kluwer Academic.

Gordon, R. M. 1987. *The Structure of Emotions: Investigations in Cognitive Philosophy*. New York: Cambridge University Press.

Greenberg, J., and S. Mitchell. 1983. *Object Relations and Psychoanalytic Theory*. Cambridge, MA: Harvard University Press.

Greenspan, P. 1988. *Emotions and Reasons: An Inquiry into Emotional Justification*. New York: Routledge.

Guarnaccia, P. J., M. Rivera, F. Franco, and C. Neighbors. 1996. Experiences of ataques de nervios: Towards an anthropology of emotions in Puerto Rico. *Culture, Medicine, and Psychiatry* 20(3):343–367.

Guralnik, D. B. ed. 1971. *Webster's New World Dictionary of the American Language*. Cleveland: World Publishing.

Habermas, J. 1971. *Knowledge and Human Interests*. Boston: Beacon Press.

Hall, J. A., T. S. Stein, D. L. Roter, and N. Resiser. 1999. Inaccuracies in physicians' perceptions of their patients. *Medical Care* 37(11):1164–1168.

Halpern, J. 1993. Empathy: Using resonance emotions in the service of curiosity. In *Empathy and the Practice of Medicine*, edited by H. Spiro and et al. New Haven: Yale University Press.

Harding, S. 1991. *Whose Science? Whose Knowledge?* Ithaca: Cornell University Press.

Harries, K. 1973. Descartes, perspective and the angelic eye. *Yale French Studies* (49):28–42.

Harrigan, J. A., J. F. Gramata, K. S. Lucic, and C. Margolis. 1989. It's how you say it: Physicians' vocal behavior. *Social Science and Medicine* 28(1):87–92.

Hegel, G. F. 1977. *Phenomenology of Spirit*. Translated by A. V. Miller. New York: Oxford University Press.

Heidegger, M. 1962. *Being and Time*. New York: Harper and Row.

Heidegger, M. 1977. The question concerning technology. In *The Question Concerning Technology and Other Essays*. New York: Harper & Row.

Heiney, S. P., J. Ruffin, and K. Goon-Johnson. 1995. The effects of a support group on selected psychosocial outcomes of bereaved parents whose child died from cancer. *Journal of Pediatric Oncology Nursing* 12(2):51–58; discussion 59–61.

Herman, B. 1993a. Mutual aid and respect for persons. In *The Practice of Moral Judgement*. Cambridge, MA: Harvard University Press.

Herman, B. 1993b. The practice of moral judgment. In *The Practice of Moral Judgment*. Cambridge, MA: Harvard University Press.

Heymann, J. 1995. *Equal Partners: A Physician's Call for a New Spirit of Medicine*. Boston: Little, Brown.

Hillman, A. L. 1998. Mediators of trust. *Journal of the American Medical Association* 280(19):1703–1704.

Hirschfeld, R., and T. Shea. 1995. Mood disorders: Psychological treatments. In *Comprehensive Textbook of Psychiatry*, edited by H. Kaplan and B. Saddock. Baltimore: Williams and Wilkins.

Holland, J. C., N. Geary, A. Marchini, and S. Tross. 1987. An international survey of physician attitudes and practice in regard to revealing the diagnosis of cancer. *Cancer Investigation* 5(2):151–154.

Hooker, W. 1849. *Physician and Patient: A Practical View of Medical Ethics*. New York: Arno Press.

Hooper, E. M., L. M. Comstock, J. M. Goodwin, and J. S. Goodwin. 1982. Patient characteristics that influence physician behavior. *Medical Care* 20:630–638.

Howell, J. 1995. *Technology in the Hospital*. Baltimore: John Hopkins University Press.

Hume, D. 1978 (1740). *A Treatise for Human Nature*. Translated by P. H. Nidditch, edited by L. A. Selby-Bigge. 2nd ed. Oxford: Oxford University Press.

Hunsdahl, J. 1967. Concerning *Einfühlung* (empathy): A conceptual analysis of its origin and early development. *Journal of the History of Behavioral Sciences* 3(2):180–191.

Husserl, E. 1977. *Cartesian Meditations: Introduction to Phenomenology*. The Hague: Martinus Nijhoff.

Jackson, S. 1990. The imagination and the psychology of healing. *Journal of the History of Behavioral Sciences* 26:345–358.

Jackson, S. 1992. The listening healer and the history of psychological healing. *The American Journal of Psychiatry* 149(12):1623–1632.

Kahneman, D., and A. Tversky. 1982. Representativeness. In *Judgement Under Uncertainty: Heuristics and Biases*, edited by D. Kahneman, P. Slovic, and A. Tversky. New York: Cambridge University Press.

Kane, F. I. 1985. Keeping Elizabeth Bouvia alive for the public good. *Hastings Center Report* 15(6):5–8.

Kant, I. 1964. *Groundwork of the Metaphysics of Morals*. Translated by H. J. Paton. New York: Harper & Row.

Kant, I. 1965. *Critique of Pure Reason*. Translated by N. K. Smith. New York: St. Martin's.

Kant, I. 1991. *Metaphysics of Morals*. New York: Cambridge University Press.

Katz, J. 1984. *The Silent World of Doctor and Patient*. New York: Free Press.

Katzenstein, M. 1987. Politics, feminism and the ethics of care. In *Women and*

Moral Theory, edited by E. F. Kittay and D. Meyers. Totowa, N.J.: Rowman and Littlefield.

Kemeny, M. E., and L. Dean. 1995. Effects of AIDS-related bereavement on HIV progression among New York City gay men. *Aids Education and Prevention* 7(5 suppl):36–47.

Klein, M. 1952. Notes on some schizoid mechanisms. In *Developments in Psychoanalysis*, edited by M. Klein, P. Heimann, S. Isaacs, and J. Riviere. London: Hogarth Press.

Kleinman, A. 1988. The personal and social meanings of illness. In *The Illness Narratives: Suffering, Healing, and the Human Condition*. New York: Basic Books.

Kleinman, A. 1995. *Writing at the Margin: Discourse Between Anthropology and Medicine*. Berkeley: University of California Press.

Kleinman, A., and B. Good, eds. 1985. *Culture and Depression: Studies in Anthropology and Cross-Cultural Psychiatry of Affect and Disorder*. Series Edit C. Leslie, *Comparative Studies of Health Systems and Medical Care*. Berkeley: University of California Press.

Kleinman, A., V. Das, and M. Lock, eds. 1997. *On Social Suffering*. Berkeley: University of California Press.

Kohut, H. 1959. Introspection, empathy and psychoanalysis. *Journal of the American Psychoanalytic Association* 7:459–483.

Kosman, L. A. 1980. Being properly affected: Virtues and feelings in Aristotle's Ethics. In *Essays on Aristotle's Ethics*, edited by A. Rorty. Berkeley: University of California Press.

Koss, M., and M. Harvey. 1991. *The Rape Victim: Clinical and Community Interventions*. 2d ed. London: Sage Publishers.

Kouyanou, K., C. E. Pither, S. Rabe-Hersketh, and S. Wessely. 1998. A comparative study of iatrogenesis, medication abuse, and psychiatric mordibity in chronic pain patients with and without medically explained symptoms. *Pain* 76(3):417–426.

Krumholz, H. M., J. Butler, J. Miller, V. Vaccarino, C. S. Williams, C. F. Mendes de Leon, T. E. Seeman, S. V. Kasl, and L. F. Berkman. 1998. Prognostic importance of emotional support for elderly patients hospitalized with heart failure. *Circulation* 97(10):958–964.

Kübler-Ross, E. 1975. *On Death and Dying*. New York: Harper & Row.

Kvale, J. L., Berg, J. Y., Groff, and G. Lange. 1999. Factors associated with resident's attitudes towards dying patients. *Family Medicine* 31(10):691–696.

Ladd, J. 1979. Legalism and medical ethics. *Journal of Medicine and Philosophy* 4:70–80.

Langer, S. 1953. *Feeling and Form: A Theory of Art*. New York: Charles Scribners' Sons.

Lantos, J. D. 1997. *Do We Still Need Doctors?* New York: Routledge.

Leake, C. D., ed. 1975. *Percival's Medical Ethics*. 2d ed. Huntington: R. E. Krieger.

Lear, J. 1988. Katharsis. *Phronesis: A Journal for Ancient Philosophy* 33:297–326.

Lear, J. 1995. *Love and Its Place in Nature*. Cambridge, MA: Harvard University Press.

Lear, J. 1998. Knowingness and abandonment: An Oedipus for our time. In *Open Minded: Working Out the Logic of the Soul*. Cambridge, MA: Harvard University Press.

Leavitt, J. 1996. Meaning and feeling in the anthropology of emotions. *American Ethnologist* 23(3):514–539.

Leslie, C., and A. Young, eds. 1992. *Paths to Asian Medical Knowledge*. Series Edit J. M. Janzen. Founding editor C. Leslie. *Comparative Studies of Health Systems and Medical Care*. Berkeley: University of California Press.

Lester, W. M., et al. 1995. Assessing the psychological types of specialists to assist students in career choice. *Academic Medicine* 70(10):932–933.

Levenson, R., and A. Ruef. 1992. Empathy: A physiological substrate. *Journal of Personality and Social Psychology* 63(2):234–246.

Levinson, W., and N. Chaumeton. 1999. Communication between surgeons and patients in routine office visits. *Surgery* 125:127–134.

Levinson, W., and D. Roter. 1995. Physicians' psychosocial beliefs correlate with their patient communication skills. *Journal of General Internal Medicine* 10:375–379.

Lifton, R. J. 1986. *The Nazi Doctors: Medical Killings and the Psychology of Genocide*. New York: Basic Books.

Lind, S., M.-J. Delvecchio Good, S. Seidel, T. Csordas, and B. J. Good. 1989. Telling the diagnosis of cancer. *Journal of Clinical Oncology* 7(5):583–589.

Linnett, L. 1988. Last impressions. In *A Piece of My Mind*, edited by B. Dan and R. Young. New York: Random House.

Lipps, T. 1935. Empathy, inner imitation and sense-feelings. In *A Modern Book of Aesthetics: An Anthology*, edited by M. Rader. New York: Henry Holt.

Lipsyte, R. 1998. The death of a brilliant surgeon who lived in the fast lane. *New York Times*; 29 March 1998. Section 1421, p. 1.

Longhurst, M. F. 1980. Angry patient, angry doctor. *Canadian Medical Assocation Journal* 123:597–598.

Lutz, C. A., and G. M. White. 1986. The anthropology of emotions. *Annual Reviews in Anthropology* 15:405–436.

Malin, A., and J. Grotstein. 1966. Projective identification in the therapeutic process. *International Journal of Psychoanalysis* 47:26–31.

Marion, R. 1988. In the back of the ambulance. In *A Piece of My Mind*, edited by B. Dan and R. Young. New York: Random House.

McKenny, G. P. 1997. *To Relieve the Human Condition: Bioethics, Technology, and the Body*. Albany: State University of New York Press.

Medical School Objectives Writing Group. 1999. Learning objectives for medical student education—guidelines for medical schools: Report I of the Medical School Objectives Project. *Academic Medicine* 74(1):13–18.

Meyers, D. 1997. *Feminists Rethink the Self.* Boulder: Westview Press.

Mills, T., and S. Kleinman. 1988. Emotions, reflexivity, and action: An interactionist analysis. *Social Forces* 66(4):1009–1027.

Mizrahi, T. 1984. Coping with patients: Subcultural adjustments to the conditions of work among internists-in-training. *Social Problems* 32(December):156–163.

More, E. and M. Milligan. 1994. *The Empathic Practitioner.* New Brunswick: Rutgers University Press.

Morse, J. M., and C. Mitcham. 1997a. Compathy: The contagion of physical distress. *Journal of Advanced Nursing* 26(4):649–657.

Morse, J. M., G. A. Havens, and S. Wilson. 1997b. The comforting interaction: Developing a model of nurse–patient relationship. *Scholarly Inquiry for Nursing Practice* 11(4):321–343; discussion 345–347.

Morse, J. M., and R. C. Intrieri. 1997c. "Talk to me": Patient communication in a long-term care facility. *Journal of Psychosocial Nursing and Mental Health Services* 35(5):34–39.

Murphy, R. 1990. *The Body Silent.* New York: Norton.

Noddings, N. 1984. *Caring: A Feminine Approach to Ethics and Moral Education.* Berkeley: University of California Press.

Novack, D., R. Plumer, R. L. Smith, H. Ochitill, G. Morrow, and J. M. Bennett. 1979. Changes in physicians' attitudes towards telling the cancer patient. *Journal of the American Medical Association* 241(9):897–900.

Nussbaum, M. 1994. *The Therapy of Desire: Theory and Practice in Hellenistic Ethics.* Princeton: Princeton University Press.

Oken, D. 1961. What to tell cancer patients: A study of medical attitudes. *Journal of the American Medical Association* 175:1120–1128.

O'Shaughnessy, B. 1980. *The Will: A Dual Aspect Theory.* Cambridge: Cambridge University Press.

Osler, W. 1963. *Aequanimitas.* New York: Norton.

Peabody, F. W. 1927. *The Care of the Patient.* Cambridge, MA: Harvard University Press.

Perrin, E. 1981. "There's a demon in your belly": Children's understanding of illness. *Pediatrics* 67(6):841–849.

Ptacek, J. T., and T. L. Eberhardt. 1996. Breaking bad news: A review of the literature. *Journal of the American Medical Association* 276(6):496–502.

Ptacek, J. T., E. A. Fries, T. L. Eberhardt, and J. J. Ptacek. 1999. Breaking bad news to patients: Physicians' perceptions of the process. *Support Care in Cancer* 7:113–120.

Quill, T. and C. Cassell. 1996. Non-abandonment: A central obligation for physicians. *Annals of Internal Medicine.* 122(5):368–374.

Rabin, S., B. Maoz, and G. Elata-Alster. 1999. Doctors' narratives in Balint groups. *British Journal of Medical Psychology* 72(1):121–125.

Racker, H. 1968. *Transference and Counter-Transference.* New York: International University Press.

Rhodes, L. A., C. A. McPhillips-Tangum, C. Markham, and R. Klenk. 1999. The power of the visible: The meaning of diagnostic tests in chronic back pain. *Social Science and Medicine* 48:1189–1203.

Rietveld, S., and P. J. M. Prins. 1998. The relationship between negative emotions and acute subjective and objective symptoms of childhood asthma. *Psychological Medicine* 1998 28(n2):407–415.

Rodriguez, M. A., H. M. Bauer, Y. Flores-Ortiz, and S. Szkupinksi-Quiroga. 1998. Factors affecting patient–physician communication for abused Latina and Asian immigrant women. *Journal of Family Practice* 47(4):309–311.

Rosch, P. J. 1987. Dealing with physician stress. *Medical Aspects of Human Sexuality* 21(4):73–93.

Rosenberg, J., and B. Towers. 1986. The practice of empathy as a prerequisite for informed consent. *Theoretical Medicine* 7 (2):181–194.

Ross, J., and J. Halpern. 1995. Ethics and geriatrics. In *The Comprehensive Textbook of Psychiatry,* edited by H. I. Kaplan and B. J. Saddock. Baltimore: Williams and Wilkins.

Roter, D., M. Stewart, S. M. Putnam, M. Lipkin, et al. 1997. Communication patterns of primary care physicians. *Journal of the American Medical Association* 277(4):350–356.

Roter, D. L., J. A. Hall, R. Merisca, B. Nordstrom, D. Cretin, and B. Svarstad. 1998. Effectiveness of interventions to improve patient compliance: A meta-analysis. *Medical Care* 36(8):1138–1161.

Ryle, G. 1949. *The Concept of Mind.* New York: Barnes & Noble.

Sarr, M. G., and A. L. Warshaw. 1999. How well do we communicate with patients as surgeons? *Surgery* 125(2):126.

Sartre, J.-P. 1956. The look. In *Being and Nothingness.* New York: Philosophical Library.

Sartre, J.-P. 1966. *Being and Nothingness.* New York: Washington Square Press.

Sartre, J.-P. 1975 (1948). *The Emotions: The Outline of a Theory.* Secaucus, New Jersey: Citadel Press.

Sawyier, F. H. 1975. A conceptual analysis of empathy. *The Annual of Psychoanalysis* 3:37–47.

Schott, R. M. 1988. *Cognition and Eros: A Critique of the Kantian Paradigm.* Boston: Beacon Press.

Schutz, A. 1967. Intersubjective understanding. In *The Phenomenology of the Social World.* Chicago: Northerwestern University Press.

Schwarzer, R., C. Dunkel-Schetter, and M. Kemeny. 1994. The multidimensional nature of received social support in gay men at risk of HIV infection and AIDS. *American Journal of Community Psychology* 22(3):319–339.

Segal, S., et al. 1996. Race, quality of care and antipsychotic prescribing practices in emergency services. *Psychiatric Services* 47(3):282–286.

Seligman, M. E. P. 1991. *Learned Optimism*. New York: A. A. Knopf.

Simpson, J. A., and E. S. C. Weiner. 1989. *The Oxford English Dictionary*. 2d ed. New York: Oxford University Press.

Sleath, B., D. L. Roter, B. Chewning, and B. Svarstad. 1999. Asking questions about medication: Analysis of physician–patient interactions and physician perceptions. *Medical Care* 37(11):1169–1173.

Smith, R. C. 1984. Teaching interviewing skills to medical students: The issue of countertransferance. *Journal of Medical Education* 59:582–588.

Sobo, E. J. 1996. Jamaican body's role in emotional experience and sense perception: Feelings, hearts, minds, and nerves. *Culture, medicine, and psychiatry* 20(3):313–342.

Solomon, R. C. 1984. Emotions and choice. In *What Is An emotion?*, edited by C. Calhoun and R. C. Solomon. Oxford: Oxford University Press.

Solomon, R. C. 1998a. Nature of emotions. In *Routledge Encyclopedia of Philosophy*, edited by E. Craig. New York: Routledge.

Solomon, R. C. 1998b. Philosophy of emotions. In *Routledge Encyclopedia of Philosophy*, edited by E. Craig. New York: Routledge.

Spiro, H., ed. 1993. *Empathy and the practice of medicine*. New Haven: Yale University Press.

Stavrakis, P. 1997. Heroic medicine, blood-letting, and the sad fate of George Washington. *Maryland Medical Journal* 46(10):539–540.

Stein, E. 1964. *On the Problem of Empathy*. The Hague: Martinus Nijhoff.

Stein, H. 1985. *The Psychodynamics of Medical Practice*. Berkeley: University of California Press.

Stein, N., S. Folkman, T. Trabasso, and T. A. Richards. 1997. Appraisal and goal processes as predictors of psychological well-being in bereaved caregivers. *Journal of Personality and Social Psychology* 72(4):872–784.

Stoller, R. J. 1985. *Observing the Erotic Imagination*. New Haven: Yale University Press.

Stolorow, R. D., et al. 1987. *Psychoanalytic Treatment: An Intersubjective Approach*: Hillsdale, NJ: Analytic Press.

Strachey, J. 1981 (1934). The nature of therapeutic action of psychoanalysis. In *Classics in Psychoanalytic Technique*, edited by R. Langs. New York: Jason Aronson.

Suchman, A., K. Markakis, H. Beckman, and R. Frankel. 1997. A model of empathic communication in the medical interview. *Journal of the American Medical Association* 277(8):678–682.

Sullivan, H. S. 1953. *The Interpersonal Theory of Psychiatry*. New York: Norton.

Sutton, M., G. E. Atweh, T. D. Cashman, and W. T. Davis. 1999. Resolving conflicts: Misconceptions and myths in the care of the patient with sickle cell disease. *Mount Sinai Journal of Medicine* 66(4):282–285.

Terr, L. 1990. *Too Scared to Cry: Psychic Trauma in Childhood*. New York: Basic Books.

Thalberg, I. 1984. Emotion and thought. In *What Is an Emotion?*, edited by C. Calhoun and R. C. Solomon. Oxford: Oxford University Press.

Theunissen, M. 1986. *The Other: Studies in the Social Ontology of Husserl, Heidegger, Sartre, and Buber*. Translated by C. Macann. Cambridge, MA: MIT Press.

Thom, D. H., and B. Cambell. 1997. Patient–physician trust: An exploratory study. *Journal of Family Practice* 44(2):169–176.

Tolstoy, L. 1981. *Death of Ivan Illych*. Translated by Solotaroff. New York: Bantam Books.

Tomkins, S. 1963. *Affect, Imagery, and Consciousness*. 2 vol. New York: Springer.

Tugendhat, E. 1986. *Self-Consciousness and Self-Determination*. Translated by P. Stern. Cambridge, MA: MIT Press.

Velleman, J. D. 1999. Love as a moral emotion. *Ethics* 109(2):338–374.

Walsh, R. A., A. Girgis, and R. W. Sanson-Fisher. 1998. Breaking bad news 2: What evidence is available to guide clinicians? *Behavioral Medicine* 24 (summer):61–72.

Williams, B. 1981. *Moral Luck*. New York: Cambridge University Press.

Williams, C. L., and R. M. Tappen. 1999. Can we create a therapeutic relationship with nursing home residents in the later stages of Alzheimer's disease? *Journal of Psychosocial Nursing* 37(3):28–35.

Wilters, J. H. 1998. Stress, burnout and physician productivity. *Medical Group Management Journal* 45(3):32–34, 36–37.

Winnicott, D. W. 1949a. Hate in the counter-transference. *International Journal of Psychoanalysis* 30(11):69–74.

Winnicott, D. W. 1965. *The Maturational Processes and the Facilitating Environment*. New York: International Universities Press.

Winnicott, D. W. 1975 (1958). Transitional objects and transitional phenomena. In *Through Paèdiatrics to Psycho-Analysis*. London: Tavistock.

Wittgenstein, L. 1958. *Philosophical Investigations*. New York: MacMillan.

Wollheim, R. 1977. Identification and imagination. In *Philosophers on Freud*, edited by R. Wollheim. New York: Jason Aronson.

Wollheim, R. 1999. *On the Emotions: The Ernst Cassirer Lectures*. New Haven: Yale University Press.

Wurzberger, B., and N. B. Levy. 1990. A "hateful epileptic" patient in the burn unit. *General Hospital Psychiatry* v. 12(n3):198–204.

Yager, T., et al. 1984. Some problems associated with war experience in men of the Vietnam generation. *Archives of General Psychiatry* 41(4):327–333.

Index